ART THERAPY WITH STUDENTS AT RISK

ABOUT THE AUTHOR

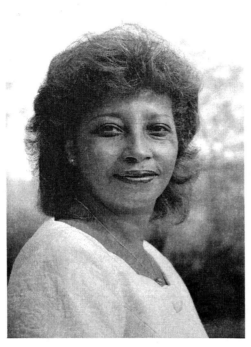

Stella A. Stepney received her B.A. degree in Art Therapy from St. Thomas Aquinas College in Sparkill, New York. She received her M.S. degree in Art Therapy from Nazareth College in Rochester, New York. She is the recipient of the Year 2000 "Award For Excellence in Art Therapy" from Nazareth College. This accolade is awarded to one student from the graduating art therapy class who has demonstrated the highest caliber for delivery of clinical services as well as academic performance. During the 1999-2000 school year, Ms. Stepney researched, planned, organized, developed, and implemented an art therapy program designed to meet the needs of at-risk students referred to the Alternative Education Department at the Monroe #1 Board of Cooperative Educational Services (BOCES) in Fairport, New York. The opportunity to design and implement an art therapy program into an alternative learning environment for adolescents laid the foundational framework for her Master's thesis. She has guest lectured in the Graduate Art Therapy Program at Nazareth College on the topic "From Thesis to Publication: Art Therapy with Students At Risk." Ms. Stepney has ten years of professional work experience in the field of Human Resources. She has teaching experience in the area of Early Childhood Education. She has designed and conducted museum tours for school-age children. A member of the American Art Therapy Association, Inc., the American Counseling Association, the Rochester Area Group Psychotherapy Society, Inc., and the Reclaiming Youth Collaborative of Rochester, Ms. Stepney resides with her husband, Harold, in Fairport, New York. They have an adult son, Terence.

ART THERAPY WITH STUDENTS AT RISK

Introducing Art Therapy into an Alternative Learning Environment for Adolescents

By

STELLA A. STEPNEY, M.S.

With a Foreword by

Ellen G. Horovitz, Ph.D., A.T.R., B.C.

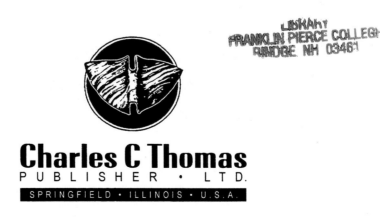

Charles C Thomas
PUBLISHER · LTD.
SPRINGFIELD · ILLINOIS · U.S.A.

Published and Distributed Throughout the World by

CHARLES C THOMAS • PUBLISHER, LTD.
2600 South First Street
Springfield, Illinois 62704

© 2001 by CHARLES C THOMAS • PUBLISHER, LTD.

ISBN 0-398-07195-0 (hard)
ISBN 0-398-07218-3 (paper)

Library of Congress Catalog Card Number: 2001027437

With THOMAS BOOKS *careful attention is given to all details of manufacturing
and design. It is the Publisher's desire to present books that are satisfactory as to their
physical qualities and artistic possibilities and appropriate for their particular use.*
THOMAS BOOKS *will be true to those laws of quality that assure a good name
and good will.*

Printed in the United States of America
MM-R-3

Photography by Harold J. Stepney

Library of Congress Cataloging-in-Publication Data

Stepney, Stella A.
    Art therapy with students at risk : introducing art therapy into an alternative learn-
ing environment for adolescents / by Stella A. Stepney ; with a foreword by Ellen G.
Horovitz.
        p.cm.
    Includes bibliographical references and index.
    ISBN 0-398-07195-0 (hard) -- ISBN 0-398-07218-3 (pbk.)
    1. Art therapy for teenagers. 2. Problem youth--Rehabilitation. I. Title.

RJ505.A7 S74 2001
616.8'5156'0835--dc21
                                                                                    2001027437

"... To Him who is able to do immeasurably more than we can ask or imagine according to His power that is within us ..."
Ephesians 3:20
NIV
and
To my husband, Harold, and my son, Terence
for your
love, support, and encouragement.

FOREWORD

Risk taking is a theme that courses through this treatise. Stella Stepney sprinkles doses of clinical acumen into this work while simultaneously offering the reader sound direction for setting up an art therapy program in an alternative high school setting. The manner in which Ms. Stepney has tackled this vast subject is both comprehensive and groundbreaking. The text covers historical and developmental overviews of art therapy programs in educational settings and outlines implementation of alternative programs, which encompass art therapy. But more importantly, Ms. Stepney covers this material in a most far-reaching manner.

Primarily, this opus begins by taking into account the physical, cognitive, moral, social, emotional, and creative development of an adolescent. Establishing this vantagepoint sets the groundwork for this sojourn. As well, Ms. Stepney's admirable compilation of these normative, developmental materials into user-friendly tables enables the viewer to look at this information contemporaneously with psychopathology as gleaned from the DSM IV-R classifications. This in itself is an extremely helpful tool in enabling the reader to organize this material into a useful platform for comparative understanding. Moreover, Ms. Stepney incorporates a glossary of psychopathic moods and affects and compares this information with developmental norms, which make these tables not only understandable but also extremely functional. The arrangement of such complex information is readily codified via Ms. Stepney's methodology and translates into discernable, usable order. This compartmentalization is a gold mine for anyone who has attempted to translate the complexities of the DSM IV-R into practical operation. But that's just the beginning.

The book then delves into everything a reader would need from establishing a rationale for instituting art therapy into an alternative school environment to types of diagnostic information to be correlated. Ms. Stepney does this with great aplomb while definitively reviewing theoretical frameworks, methodologies, and assessment batteries from a variety of sources. While these are then translated into art therapy techniques, Ms. Stepney tailors the aforementioned directives and modifies previous researchers' ideas with ideas of her own. This is done rather meticulously and is then introduced into case vignettes so that the reader can witness firsthand how such contemplation could be configured into such an alternative educational environment.

Ms. Stepney seems to have thought of everything from IDEA '97 (Individuals with Disabilities Education Act) to partnering successfully within an educational environment and establishing the most comprehensive release form I have seen designed to date. No stone was left unturned in this complete referendum. Anyone who wants to bring art therapy to the schools must have this compendium. It is a must. Art Therapy and Art Education have been dually wedded in this incredible weave. May the tapestry unfold as art therapists forge into this educational domain, weave together the tattered threads of an alternative existence, and minister these underserved youth into health.

Ellen G. Horovitz, Ph.D., A.T.R., B.C.
Director of Graduate Art Therapy
Nazareth College
Rochester, New York

PREFACE

At the beginning of the twentieth century, education reformers made eloquent pleas for the education of the "whole" child—the social, emotional, physical, cognitive, and creative components. Since students are educated by means of the environment in the twenty-first century, special consideration must be given to the design of both traditional and nontraditional learning environments.

Adolescents who are referred to alternative learning environments are considered to be students who are at risk with the potential for displaying academic, behavioral, and social problems. Academically at-risk students fail to achieve and are predictably dropout prone. Behaviorally at-risk students display inappropriate school behaviors. Socially at-risk students are faced with disciplinary charges and may have been brought to the attention of the juvenile justice system. Researchers have isolated factors that describe the attitudes and personality characteristics of students who are at risk. These factors include defensiveness and hopelessness, attention-seeking, antisocial disorders, conduct disorders, interpersonal problems, and family relationship problems.

Researchers suggest that professionals designing alternative education programs should consider both the at-risk factors and the attitudes and personality characteristics of students in order to develop effective interventions. They recommend that effective school programs should include intensive individual and group counseling focusing on self-esteem, self-concept, personal responsibility, and the appropriate expression of feelings. Students who are at risk must be convinced of their own self-worth and be able to foresee the consequences of the choices they make.

Art therapy, in an educational setting, is a psychoeducational therapeutic intervention that focuses upon art media as primary expressive and communicative channels. The art therapy process allows students to explore personal problems and potentials and find ways of making responsible choices.

Research points out that many students currently placed in alternative school programs would qualify for special educational services following psychological evaluation. The Education for All Handicapped Children Act of 1975, Public Law 94-142, in its original form, identified art therapy as a viable service that could benefit a student who required special education. Public Law 94-142 made it possible for school systems to allocate monies to help fund art therapy. However, it should be noted that students who are not identified as disabled but who experience difficulty in school as a result of academic, behavioral, and social problems could also benefit from art therapy.

This book represents the research, planning, organization, development, and implementation of an art therapy program into an alternative learning environment. It is designed for graduate art therapy students, professional art therapists, educators, counselors, school psychologists, social workers, and individuals interested in the application of art therapy.

The book is divided into six chapters. Unique to this resource is the inclusion of 14 art therapy techniques, written using a lesson plan format, that have proven to bridge not only the verbal and nonverbal, but also the logical and emotional. Photographic illustrations highlight the students' creative responses to the techniques.

Chapter 1, *Adolescence*, examines the developmental period of adolescence. The physical, cognitive, moral, social, emotional, and creative components are discussed. This period is characterized by challenges. From a developmental perspective, disordered behavior is viewed as a developmental deviation. Precursors of later disorders are looked for within the challenges that are most notable. If development is amiss in these critical areas, there is the potential for further problems.

Chapter 2, *Alternative Schools*, traces the evolution of the alternative schools movement from the Civil Rights Movement of the 1960s to the present. Mary Anne Raywid is recognized as a leading contemporary advocate for alternative schools. Raywid emphasizes that from their inception, alternative schools have been designed to "respond to a group that appears not to be optimally served by the regular program." Consequently, alternative schools have represented varying degrees of departure from standard school organization, programs, and environment. The three "pure" types of alternative schools are highlighted.

Chapter 3, *Alternative Education Programs*, explores the dual catalysts for policymakers to embrace alternative education. These catalysts are the desire to increase graduation rates and the need to eliminate disruptive or violent students from the classroom without sending them into the streets. The Alternative Education Department of Monroe #1 Board of Cooperative Educational Services (BOCES) in Fairport, New York was officially formed in July of 1998. This department, under the administration of David R. Halpern, is a progressive alternative learning environment that possesses the characteristics of innovation, autonomy, and empowerment that have contributed to the overall success of the students referred to the programs.

Chapter 4, *Emotions and Learning*, provides insight into the psychobiology of emotion and its impact on learning. Developments in the cognitive sciences have uncovered how and where the body and brain process emotion. Since emotion can be a more powerful determinant of behavior than the brain's logical or rational processes, researchers recommend that educators should develop a basic understanding of the psychobiology of emotion to enable them to evaluate emerging educational applications.

Chapter 5, *Art Therapy in the Schools*, focuses on the field of school art therapy. Janet Bush is a leading advocate for this specialization within the art therapy profession. Bush raises the question, "Will art therapy eventually be well established in all school systems and will it serve as one accepted means of addressing student failure in the classroom?" She highlights the variety of tasks that must be accomplished to make art therapy an integral part of the educational program.

Chapter 6, *Implementation of the Art Therapy Program*, presents an effective proposal for the introduction and implementation of a viable art therapy program within an alternative learning environment.

It is my hope that this book will provide practitioners with valuable insights into this unique population of students and offer intervention strategies that will lead students at risk to creative self-expression and ultimately into cognitive, social, and emotional growth.

STELLA A. STEPNEY

ACKNOWLEDGMENTS

Inspiration is defined as the stimulation of the mind or emotion to a high level of feeling or activity. Individuals who inspire stimulate creativity or action in others. During my inspirational journey, many sincere, dedicated, and committed individuals have inspired me. I would like to take this opportunity to acknowledge and thank the educators, practitioners, mentors, role models, students, friends, and family who, in their own unique way, have enabled me to make this contribution to the field of Art Therapy.

I am deeply indebted to Sister Elizabeth Slinker, OP, A.T.R. and Carol Greiff Lagstein, C.S.W., A.T.R., B.C., Director of Art Therapy, for introducing me to the profession. My undergraduate work at St. Thomas Aquinas College provided me with an understanding of the creative art therapies and how the creative process can be a pathway to greater self-awareness and self-healing.

I am appreciative of the opportunity to obtain my Master's degree from Nazareth College. I want to gratefully acknowledge Dr. Ellen G. Horovitz, A.T.R., B.C., Director of the Graduate Art Therapy Program. As an educator, Dr. Horovitz has contributed her professional knowledge, expertise, and clinical experience. As a mentor, she challenges students to enhance their therapeutic work by delving deeper into their own personal issues and exploring them fully. Dr. Horovitz has provided me with invaluable support and encouragement in reinforcing my professional capabilities. To Dr. Horovitz, Victoria Laneri, A.T.R., Sandra Ticen, A.T.R., and the Graduate Art Therapy staff at Nazareth College, thank you for providing the highest level of professional training and development that is required for art therapy students to become skilled practitioners.

I want to acknowledge and thank David R. Halpern, principal of the Alternative Education Department of Monroe #1 BOCES, for his recognition of the value of art therapy in the lives of students who are at risk. The situations, experiences, and data obtained through the introduction and implementation of the art therapy program laid the foundational framework that supports this book. To David Halpern, Dr. Tom Cascini, and the Alternative Education Department staff, thank you for your assistance and encouragement in this endeavor. Special thanks are extended to the students and their families for permitting me to include the photographic illustrations of the artwork.

A special word of appreciation goes to a dear friend, Jill Penaloza, A.T.R., B.C., for offering wise and insightful counsel.

My heartfelt thanks to a remarkable woman, Stella Wiley, for her true friendship and her moral and spiritual support.

I have been blessed with a loving and supportive family. To my aunt, Bertha Douglas, a steadfast woman of faith, thank you for role modeling graciousness, dignity, and charm under all circumstances.

To my husband, Harold, thank you for continually being the "wind beneath my wings."

"But they that wait upon the LORD shall renew *their* strength;
they shall mount up with wings as eagles;
they shall run, and not be weary;
and they shall walk, and not faint."
Isaiah 40:31
KJV

INTRODUCTION

Image-making, as a vehicle for creative self-expression or giving vent in constructive form to feelings, emotions, and thoughts at one's own level, enables us to understand and to learn. Through the process, our consciousness of the self, others, and the environment is enhanced. Carl Jung theorized that there are four functions of consciousness: sensation, intuition, feeling, and thinking. Sensation and intuition are the two functions by which "facts" and the "fact-world" is apprehended. Feeling and thinking are the two functions that judge and evaluate. In other words, we experience our world through sensation and intuition; we judge and evaluate our world through thinking and feeling. Jung (1971) explains:

> The only things we experience immediately are the contents of consciousness. . . . Consciousness seems to stream into us from outside in the form of sense perceptions. We see, hear, taste, touch, and smell the world, and so we are conscious of the world. Sense perceptions tell us that something is. But sense perceptions do not tell us what it is. . . . What it is, is told to us by the process of apperception. . . . This recognition derives from the process of thinking. Thinking tells us what a thing is. . . . The recognized image arouses emotional reactions of a pleasant or unpleasant nature, and the memory-images thus stimulated bring with them concomitant emotional phenomena which are known as feeling-tones. In this way, an object appears to us as pleasant, desirable, and beautiful, or as unpleasant, disgusting and ugly. This process is called feeling. The intuitive process is conceived as perception of the possibilities inherent in a situation. (pp. 23–26)

One definition for image is a mental picture of something not real or present. Images, as mental pictures, are universal phenomena. They are occurrences or facts that are perceptible by the senses; so they belong to the function of sensation. We experience images or mental pictures with feeling-tones, through dreams, music, poetry, and encountering scents. Therefore, image-making is the process of giving form to mental pictures with feeling-tones.

Creative power is one of the definitions for imagination. Pat Allen

(1995) explains:

> Our imagination is the most important faculty we possess. . . . It is
> through our imagination that we discern possibilities and options. A rela-
> tionship with our imagination is a relationship with our deepest self.
> Whether we have cultivated our imagination or not, we each have a lifetime
> of patterns and habits of thought embedded there based on past experi-
> ences. Our expectations of ourselves and the world flow from these patterns.
> (p. 3)

Imagination, as creative power must be "cultivated." Creative
power must be formed and refined in order to gain insight into possibilities and options. Jung (1971) points out, "It is the function of the
conscious not only to recognize and assimilate the external world
through the gateway of the senses, but to translate into visible reality,
the world within us" (p. 46).

This "world within us" can be translated into "visible reality"
through the processes inherent in drawing, painting, and sculpture. We
make visible our kinetic energy through drawing. We make visible our
sensual energy through painting. We make visible our emotional energy through color. We make visible the three-dimensional and instinc-
tual components of our experiences through sculpture.

I hear and I forget

I see and I remember

I do and I understand

In the doing is the learning

(Ancient Chinese Proverb)

REFERENCES

Allen, P. B. (1995). *Art is a Way of Knowing: A guide to self-knowledge and spiritual fulfillment through creativity.* Boston: Shambhala Publications, Inc.

Campbell, J. (Ed.). (1971). *The Portable Jung.* Translated by R. F. C. Hall. New York:
The Viking Press, Inc.

Kramer, E. (1993). *Art as Therapy with Children* (2nd ed.). Chicago: Magnolia Street
Publishers.

CONTENTS

ART THERAPY WITH STUDENTS AT RISK

Chapter 1

ADOLESCENCE

D EVELOPMENT IS DEFINED as the process of orderly, cumulative, directional, age-related changes in a person. Pathology is defined as any marked deviation from a normal, healthy state. Developmental psychopathology is the study of developmental challenges and vulnerabilities of healthy and unhealthy psychological adaptations and of the complex influences that determine developmental outcomes. Studying psychopathology, from a developmental perspective, views disordered behavior as a developmental deviation. Therefore, we must look for the precursors of later disorders within the cognitive, social, and emotional challenges that are most notable at a given age. If development is amiss in these critical areas, there is the potential for future problems.

PHYSICAL DEVELOPMENT

Adolescence is the period of growth from puberty to maturity, age 12–19 years. It is a transition period that has always been characterized by challenges. With respect to physical development, a stepped-up production of sex hormones late in middle childhood brings about the beginning of adolescence or puberty. Puberty is the period during which a child changes from a sexually immature individual to one who is capable of reproduction. Sexual maturation is accompanied by the development of secondary sex characteristics. These are noticeable transformations, which differentiate males from females but are not essential to reproduction.

COGNITIVE DEVELOPMENT

Jean Piaget (1896–1980), a Swiss biologist and pioneer in the field of developmental psychology argued that there are major qualitative changes in the way children understand and learn about the world. In Piaget's theory of cognitive development, the emphasis is on the qualitative changes (transformations) in the way children think through a series of stages in which cognition becomes less egocentric and experiential and more analytical.

There are three major cognitive advances in adolescence. Logical thinking is now applied to the possible (what might exist), not just to the real (what does exist–concrete thinking). The use of Hypothetico-Deductive Reasoning allows an adolescent to think-up hypothetical solutions to a problem (ideas about what might be) and then formulate a logical and systematic plan for deducing which of these possible solutions is the right one. In situations that require thinking about possible consequences of various courses of action, hypothetico-deductive reasoning is also useful. The ability to think about relationships among mentally constructed concepts is a cognitive advance. These are the abstract concepts built up from the more concrete things adolescents perceive.

In general, adolescents are able to reflect on the thought processes through which they gain knowledge. They are now able to think about thinking. They also have a more mature grasp of abstract concepts such as identity, justice, religion, society, existence, morality, and friendship. Piaget (1972) viewed the new thinking skills of adolescents as the product of new kinds of mental transformations. He labeled these qualitative changes Formal Operations.

Another change related to cognitive development is Adolescent Egocentrism. Egocentrism is the failure to differentiate the perspective of others from one's own point of view. Since adolescents are now able to think about their own thinking and consider abstract possibilities, they develop a new kind of egocentrism. David Elkind (1967), in describing adolescent egocentrism, stresses the concepts of Imaginary Audience and Personal Fables. An Imaginary Audience is a manifestation of adolescent egocentrism in which the young person displays an unjustified belief that he or she is the focus of other people's attention. Because adolescents can think about the thoughts of others, they are able to consider what others might be thinking of them. A Personal Fable is a manifestation of adolescent egocentrism in which the young person believes in his or her uniqueness to the point where he or she thinks that no one else has ever had his or her special thoughts and feelings.

MORAL DEVELOPMENT

Moral Reasoning is the process of thinking and making judgments about the right course of action in a given situation. Piaget (1932, 1965) included the development of moral reasoning within his theory of cognitive development. Lawrence Kohlberg (1958, 1969) developed a six-stage model of how moral reasoning changes. In Kohlberg's stage theory, most adolescents reach the period of Conventional Morality (stages 3 & 4) in which their moral judgments are based on internalized standards arising from concrete experiences in the social world. Kohlberg calls the reasoning conventional because it focuses either on the opinions of others or formal laws. In Stage 3, referred to as the "Good-Boy, Good-Girl Orientation," the young person's goal is to act in ways in which others will approve of. Actions are motivated by a fear of either actual or hypothetical disapproval than by a fear of punishment. In Stage 4, referred to as "Authority, or Law-and-Order Orientation," the basis of moral judgments shifts to concern over doing one's duty as prescribed by society's laws. Concerns about possible dishonor or concrete harm to others replace concerns about other's disapproval.

SOCIAL AND EMOTIONAL DEVELOPMENT

The developmental stage theories postulated by Sigmund Freud and Erik Erikson address the social and emotional development in adolescence. Freud developed the theory that abnormal behavior results from the inadequate expression of drives or intense urges based on human biology. According to Freud's (1966) early theory, there is only one motive that governs behavior. This motive is the satisfaction of biological needs, which in turn discharges tension. The critical component is the amount of gratification or frustration that the child experiences as he or she seeks to discharge this tension. Freud's stages of psychosexual development are defined in terms of the primary body organ used to discharge tension at each particular period of development. Faulty development can occur because of frustration at a particular psychosexual stage. This frustration can result in fixation. Fixation is the failure to progress normally through the psychosexual stages of development as a result of becoming locked into one particular psychological mode and arena of conflict, which causes the individual to express it in symbolic ways.

Psychosexual Development in Adolescence		
Age	*Stage*	*Resolution*
12–18 years	Genital	If successful: Full and satisfying genital potency; consolidation of prior accomplishments. If unsuccessful: Impaired ability to love and work; neurotic disorders.

Neo-Freudians replaced the primary focus on tension discharge with a new focus on the EGO or SELF. It is considered a more independent force, which allows individuals to be purposeful and active in mastering their experiences. Neo-Freudians think in terms of broader issues and conflicts faced from infancy through adulthood. Erik Erikson (1963) represents this new approach. In his psychosocial theory, Erikson proposes a series of developmental tasks that all people face and resolve in the same way.

Psychosocial Development in Adolescence		
Age	*Stage*	*Developmental Tasks / Issues*
12–20 years	Identity vs. Role Confusion	If successful: Adolescents build on earlier experiences to develop a sense of self-identity, particularly in relation to society. If unsuccessful: Failure to reach this goal may cause confusion in identity, the choice of an occupation, and the roles they perform as adults.

With respect to the overall social and emotional development in adolescence, adolescents must achieve a personal identity. According to L. Alan Sroufe, Robert Cooper, and Ganie Dehart (1992):

> The concept of identity includes the quest for personal discovery, the resulting sense of "who I am" and the growing understanding of the "meaning" of one's existence. Identity also involves integrating into a coherent whole one's past experiences, one's ongoing personal changes, and society's demands and expectations for one's future. (p. 519)

In Erikson's theory, the difficulty that the adolescent faces when trying to establish his or her personal identity is referred to as an identity crisis.

In addition to achieving a personal identity, Sroufe, Cooper, and DeHart (1992) identify four critical tasks of adolescence:

1. Adolescents must evolve a new understanding of the self as cohesive, integrated, and continuous, recognizing that various parts of the self are part of a whole and that different ways of behaving with different people are sensible rather than inconsistent. (Harter, 1990)
2. Adolescents must achieve a new level of closeness and trust with peers. Often this is accomplished first with peers of the same gender before moving on to intimate cross-gender relationships. (Hartup and Laursen, in press)
3. Adolescents must acquire a new status in the family. Relationships with parents become more equal as the young person grows more independent and responsible. Family ties are not severed; connections with parents merely take a different form. (Grotevant, in press)
4. Adolescents must move toward a more autonomous stance with respect to the larger world. This includes anticipating future roles, making career choices, and committing themselves to certain values. . . . This process must entail decisions that the adolescents themselves make and then actively translate into practice. (p. 518)

CREATIVE DEVELOPMENT

The two creative developmental periods are referred to as the Pseudo-Naturalistic Stage, Twelve–Fourteen Years and Adolescent Art, Fourteen–Seventeen Years: The Period of Decision. During the Period of Decision, adolescents are self-critical, introspective, and have a growing concern about their relationship to society. Art should provide the opportunity for adolescents to express feelings and emotions and to feel that their art is important to themselves and to others. Art might be considered a metaphor, or speaking to issues. It is a record of reaction and/or a record of interpretation.

Adolescents are no longer drawing and painting spontaneously; a deepened awareness of the environment, a more acute sense of SELF, and a purpose in creating becomes evident.

REFERENCES

American Psychiatric Association. (1994). *Diagnostic and Statistical Manual of Mental Disorders* (4th ed.). Washington, DC: American Psychiatric Association.

Blum, B., & Blum, G. (1986). *Feeling Good about Yourself: A Guide for People Working with People who have Disabilities or Low Self-esteem.* Mill Valley, CA: Academic Therapy Publications.

Elkind, D. (1967). Egocentrism in Adolescence. *Child Development,* 38, 1025–1034.

Erikson, E. (1963). *Childhood and Society* (2nd ed.). New York: W.W. Norton & Company.

Freud, S. (1966). *Introductory Lectures on Psychoanalysis.* J. Strochey (Ed. and Trans.). New York: W.W. Norton & Company.

Grotevant, H. (in press). Assigned and chosen identity components: A process perspective on their integration. In G. Adams, R. Montemayor, & T. Gulotta (Eds.), *Advances in Adolescent Development, 4.* Newbury Park, CA: Sage.

Harter, S. (1990). Self and identity development. In S. Feldman & G. Elliot (Eds.), *At the threshold: The Developing Adolescent* (pp. 352–387). Cambridge, MA: Harvard University Press.

Hartup, W., & Laursen, B. (in press). Conflict and context in peer relations. In C. Hart (Ed.), *Children on playgrounds: Research perspectives and applications.* Ithaca: State University of New York Press.

Kohlberg, L. (1969). Stage and sequence: The cognitive-development approach to socialization. In D. A. Goslin (Ed.), *Handbook of socialization theory and research.* Chicago: Rand McNally.

Lowenfeld, V., & Brittain, W. L. (1987). *Creative and Mental Growth* (8th ed.). New York: Macmillan Publishing Company.

Marcia, J. (1980). Identity in adolescence. In J. Adelson (Ed.), *Handbook of Adolescent Psychology,* 159–187. New York: John Wiley & Sons, Inc.

Piaget, J. (1932, 1965). *The Moral Judgment of the Child.* New York: The Free Press.

Piaget, J. (1972). Intellectual Evolution From Adolescence to Adulthood. *Human Development, 15,* 1–12.

Samuels, S. C. (1977). *Enhancing Self-Concepts in Early Childhood.* New York: Human Sciences Press.

Sroufe, L. A., Cooper, R. G., & DeHart, G. B. (1992). *Child Development: Its Nature and Course* (2nd ed.). New York: McGraw-Hill, Inc.

Chapter 2

ALTERNATIVE SCHOOLS

HISTORICAL OVERVIEW

MARIO D. FANTINI, ONE OF THE NATION'S best-known educational reformers, is recognized as a leading spokesperson for increasing educational options for students, parents, and teachers within the public schools. In the article, *"The What, Why, and Where of the Alternative Movement,"* Dr. Fantini presents a historical overview which highlights some of the pioneer educational experiments both outside and inside the public education system. Fantini (1976) points out that the evolution of the alternative schools movement can be traced back to the Civil Rights movement of the 1960s. Fantini explains:

> As the quest for desegregation gained momentum, parent, teacher, and community boycotts of public schools led to the establishment of temporary freedom schools in storefronts and church basements. Teachers, community residents, parents, and college volunteers collaborated to continue the education of black children in the "freedom schools." For many blacks and whites alike, the freedom schools provided a glimpse of alternative programs tailored to their perceived needs, which included sympathetic adults working with children, curriculum specifically geared to the self-determination concerns of black people, and involvement in the immediate political life of the community. To pursue these educational concerns, those involved departed from established procedures by assuming a flexible stance that advocated expanding the boundaries of schooling to include the community and its resources, establishing smaller educational units to humanize the experience for those involved, and relating educational experience to the life of the community. These ingredients remain prevalent in the current alternative schools movement.

The concept of "freedom schools" according to Fantini relates to being free from the bureaucracy of massive public schools. Momentum was gained through the dedication of staff and parents.

Fantini (1976) asserts:

> The important point is that there is flexibility about these schools that
> represents a refreshing departure from the uniformity of public schools. Yet
> despite their aspirations of love, independence, self-direction, tolerance, and
> social responsiveness, their real impact . . . has not been to achieve radical
> reform outside the system of public schools; but rather to stimulate a more
> progressive . . . reform effort within the public school system.

Robert Arnove and Toby Strout (1978) point out that as early as
1973, influential spokespersons such as Dr. Fantini were referring to
the alternatives as "public schools of choice" or "options within public
schooling." The authors explain, "Private alternatives defined themselves as free schools, street academies, and freedom or community
schools. The new public taxonomy included these nomenclatures:
open schools, schools-without-walls, schools-within schools, continua-
tion centers, learning centers, and multicultural schools."

TYPES OF ALTERNATIVE PROGRAMS

Mary Anne Raywid, Professor of Education, Administration and
Policy Studies at Hofstra University, is recognized as a leading contemporary advocate for alternative schools. In an article entitled,
"*Alternative Schools: The State of the Art,*" Raywid (1994) highlights the
fact that the early alternative schools like today's alternative schools
represent innovation in terms of their small scale, informal ambiance,
and departure from bureaucratic rules and procedures. Raywid (1994)
explains:

> Two enduring consistencies have characterized alternative schools from
> the start: they have been designed to respond to a group that appears not to
> be optimally served by the regular program, and consequently they have
> represented varying degrees of departure from standard school organiza-
> tion, programs, and environments.

Raywid emphasizes that the first enduring consistency has associated alternative schools with unsuccessful students, the disadvantaged,
marginal, at risk, or those who cannot or will not succeed in a regular
program. The second enduring consistency has associated alternatives
to innovation and creativity in both organization and practice.
Raywid (1994) has identified three "pure" types which individual
alternative programs approximate to varying degrees. Type I alterna-

tives are popular innovations characterized by choice. Their goal is to make school challenging and fulfilling for all individuals involved. They reflect organizational and administrative departures from the traditional, in addition to programmatic innovations. Type II alternatives are last chance programs to which students are sentenced. They are considered as one last chance prior to expulsion. These alternatives include in-school suspension programs, cool-out rooms, and longer term placement for the chronically disruptive. The primary goal is behavior modification. Type III alternatives have a remedial focus and are characterized by referral. They are offered to students who are presumed to need remediation or rehabilitation—academic, social/emotional, or both. Raywid contends that alternative schools can be identified as one of these three types, but particular programs can be a mixture of the three types. Raywid (1994) points out:

> The genre determines an alternative school's most formative features. It determines the grounds upon which the school will be evaluated; whether student affiliation is by choice, sentence, or referral; and perhaps most fundamentally, what is assumed about school and students. Both Type II and Type III set out to fix the student on the assumption that the problems lie within the individual. Type I assumes that the school-student match may explain difficulties, and that by altering a school's program and environment, one can alter student response, performance and achievement. It is this assumption that calls for responsibilities, hence school creativity.

Raywid (1994) highlights the fact that, "A fine line divides at risk or special-needs students from the rest." These terms are being applied to substantial majorities of students in all the nations urban school districts. This may be the reason why cities have taken away the lead in innovation from suburban school districts. Raywid points out, "A changing population makes new sorts of schools imperative. More challenging students are just more dependent on a good education."

STUDENTS AT RISK

Cheryl Lange (1998) emphasizes that more and more students are labeled at risk in educational systems. Lange states:

> These students are often behind academically, have dropped out of schools, or have been expelled or suspended from conventional high schools. Some states have implemented school choice options that address the needs of these students giving them a choice of an alternative high school setting.

Lange (1998) cites findings from previous studies that indicate that special education students are often enrolling in alternative schools. A 1990 survey of Minnesota's alternative schools and area learning centers conducted by Gorney & Ysseldyke (1993) found that approximately 19% of students enrolled in these programs had a disability. Of this group of students, over 50% were identified as having an emotional behavioral disorder. Lange (1998) contends:

> We know that students with disabilities are at high risk of not completing school, but we are less sure of how to address their needs. Data from this study suggest that students with disabilities are accessing the alternative programs, though many programs do not formally identify students with disabilities.

Carole G. Fuller and David A. Sabatino (1996) define at-risk students as those with the potential for displaying academic, behavioral, and social problems. The authors explain:

> Academically at-risk students fail to achieve and are predictably dropout prone. Behaviorally at-risk students display inappropriate school behaviors, while the socially at risk are faced with school disciplinary charges and may have been brought to the attention of the juvenile justice system. The development of alternative school programs was intended to provide at-risk students the opportunity to avoid academic and social failure and to prevent students from dropping out of school or becoming adjudicated.

Fuller and Sabatino (1996) cite Harl Douglass (1969) who has identified nine factors representing at-risk students:

> The factors are: (1) records of poor academic achievement, (2) family backgrounds of low socioeconomic and cultural status, (3) poor school achievement after several social promotions, (4) truancy, (5) no membership in school extracurricular activities, (6) verbal abilities inferior to nonverbal abilities, (7) records of repeated norm-violating disruptive behaviors, (8) a peer group composed of similar students, and (9) a negative attitude toward school.

Fuller and Sabatino (1996) studied selected demographic and personality characteristics in a population of 50 at-risk junior and senior high school students in four alternative schools. The authors contend that, "At-risk students are placed into alternative schools on the basis of observable behaviors, while psychological or other diagnostic procedures are not required for placement. Therefore, the presence of emotional disturbances requiring special education services go undetected."

In the 1996 Fuller and Sabatino study, the research subjects consisted of 37 male and 13 female students with a mean age of 15.1 years. The average grade level was 8.6, which indicates an age to grade level discrepancy of at least one academic year. The research measures utilized for the study were:

1. A demographic questionnaire designed with a forced option format.
2. The Minnesota Multiphasic Personality Inventory-Adolescent (MMPI-A). The MMPI-A is a true/false objective personality test for adolescents age 14–18 years.
3. The Behavior Assessment System for Children (BASC) Self-Report Form A. The BASC is a true/false objective personality test for adolescents age 12–18 years.

The MMPI-A and the BASC establish the presence of mental disorders as described in the DSM-IV and employ a self-report format.

Fuller and Sabatino's (1996) research results of the selected demographic findings indicated: (1) 82% of the subjects were Caucasian, (2) 50% endorsed no religious orientation, (3) 62% reported they received letter grades of C, D, or F on grade reports, (4) the importance of need to achieve academically, demonstrating competitive success was absent, (5) 42% indicated that they did not participate in any extracurricular activities, (6) 24% reported they were undecided about plans after high school, (7) 44% reported living in single-parent homes, and (8) 84% reported parents having completed the minimum of a high school education. The alternative school students in this sample reflected five of Douglass' (1969) nine at-risk factors: (1) poor achievement (grades) in school, (2) truancy, (3) no participation in extracurricular activities, (4) records of repeated norm violating behaviors, and (5) a negative attitude toward school.

ATTITUDES AND PERSONALITY CHARACTERISTICS OF STUDENTS AT RISK

The data obtained from the two personality tests provided a description of the attitudes and personality characteristics of alternative school students. Factor analysis of the two personality tests isolated six factors: (1) defensiveness/hopelessness, (2) attention seeking, (3) antisocial disorders, (4) conduct disorders, (5) interpersonal problems, and (6) family relationship problems. Fuller and Sabatino

(1996) contend:

> These factors portray the alternative school population as cynical, suf-
> fering academic and behavioral adjustment problems in school, possessing
> antisocial attitudes and behaviors, lacking education and/or career goals,
> and having problematic relationships with both family and peers. Also
> prominent in this description is the endorsed use/abuse of alcohol/drugs,
> which was also indicated by the results from the two personality tests.

For the relevance of the study, Fuller and Sabatino (1996) suggest
that the professionals designing alternative school programs should
consider both the at-risk factors (demographic characteristics) and personality characteristics of these students in order to develop effective
interventions. The authors make the following recommendations:

> Given the personality characteristics of this group, the need for individ-
> ual psychological assessment of each student entering an alternative pro-
> gram becomes apparent. Many students currently placed into alternative
> school programs would qualify for special education services following psy-
> chological evaluation. Some would be learning disabled, some seriously
> emotionally disturbed, and some comorbid with both conditions. To be
> effective, alternative school programs should include intensive individual
> and group counseling focusing on self-esteem, self-concept, personal
> responsibility, appropriate expression of feelings, drug/alcohol prevention,
> vocational assessment, and career exploration and preparation. Family
> counseling could be an integral phase of treatment if the participation of the
> parents/caregivers is obtained. These students must be convinced of their
> own self-worth and be able to foresee the consequences of the choices they
> make.

REFERENCES

American Psychiatric Association. (1994). *Diagnostic and Statistical Manual of Mental
Disorders* (4th ed.). Washington, DC: American Psychiatric Association.
Arnove, R., & Strout T. (1978). Alternative Schools and Cultural Pluralism: Promise
and Reality. *Educational Research Quarterly*, Vol. 2, No. 4, 74–95.
Brendtro, L. K., Brokenleg, M., & Van Bockern, S. (1990). *Reclaiming Youth At-Risk:
Our Hope for the Future.* Bloomington, IN: National Educational Services.
Coopersmith, S. (1967). *The Antecedents of Self-esteem.* San Francisco, CA: W. H.
Freeman and Company.
Douglass, H. R. (1969). An Effective Junior High School Program for Reducing the
Number of Dropouts. *Contemporary Education*, Vol. 41, 34–37.
Fantini, M. (Ed.) (1976). *Alternative Education: A Source Book for Parents, Teachers,
Students, and Administrators.* Garden City, NY: Anchor Books.
Fuller, C. G. & Sabatino, D. A. (1996). Who Attends Alternative High Schools? *The*

High School Journal, Vol. 79, No. 4, 293–297.

Garrison, R. (1987). *Alternative Schools for Disruptive Youth.* Malibu, CA: National School Safety Center, Pepperdine University.

Gorney, D. J., & Ysseldyke, J. E. (1993). Students with Disabilities Use of Various Options to Access Alternative Schools and Area Learning Centers. *Special Services in Schools*, Vol. 7, 124–143.

Gray, M. E. (1988). *Images: A Workbook for Enhancing Self-esteem and Promoting Career Preparation, Especially for Black Girls.* Sacramento, CA: California Department of Education.

Hurst, D. S. (1994). We Cannot Ignore the Alternatives. *Educational Leadership*, Vol. 52, No. 1, 78–79.

Lange, C. M. (1998). Characteristics of Alternative Schools and Programs Serving At-Risk Students. *The High School Journal*, Vol. 81, No. 4, 183–198.

Lichter, S. O., Rapien, E. B., Seibert, F. M., & Morris, A. (1962). *The Drop-Outs: A Treatment Study of Intellectually Capable Students Who Drop Out of High School.* New York: The Free Press of Glencoe.

Maxmen, J. S., & Ward, N. G. (1995). *Essential Psychopathology and Its Treatment* (2nd edition Revised for DSM-IV). New York: W. W. Norton & Company.

Mesinger, J. F. (1982). Alternative Education for Behavior Disordered and Delinquent Adolescent Youth: What Works–Maybe? *Behavioral Disorders: Journal of the Council for Children with Behavioral Disorders*, Vol. 7, No. 2, 91–100.

OERI Goal 2 Work Group. (1993). *Reaching the Goals, Goal 2: High School Completion.* Washington, DC: Office of Educational Research and Improvement, U.S. Department of Education.

Piotrowski, C., Sherry, D., & Keller, J. W. (1985). Psychodiagnostic Test Usage: A Survey of the Society for Personality Assessment. *Journal of Personality Assessment*, Vol. 49, 115–119.

Radin, N. (1988). Alternatives to Suspension and Corporal Punishment. *Urban Education*, Vol. 22, No. 4, 476–495.

Raywid, M. A. (1994). Alternative Schools: The State of the Art. *Educational Leadership*, Vol. 52, No. 1, 26–31.

Reynolds, C., & Kamphaus, R. (1992). *Behavior Assessment System for Children Manual.* Circle Pines, MN: American Guidance Services, Inc.

Scherer, M. (1994). On Schools Where Students Want to Be: A Conversation with Deborah Meier. *Educational Leadership*, Vol. 52, No. 1, 4–8.

Stevens, C. J., Tullis, R. J., Sanchez, K. S., & Gonzalez, J. (1991). *An Evaluation of the Alternative Schools 1990–91.* Houston, TX: Houston Independent School District, Texas Department of Research and Evaluation.

Streva, M. A. (1983). The Evolution of Discipline: Alternative to Suspension Programs. Presented in partial fulfillment of requirements for Education 598, New Mexico State University.

Sylwester, R. (1994). How Emotions Affect Learning. *Educational Leadership*, Vol. 52, No. 2, 60–65.

Weiner, R. (1985). *P. L. 94-142: Impact on the Schools.* Arlington, VA: Capitol Publications Inc.

Williams, C., Butcher, J., Ben-Porath, Y, & Graham, J. (1992). *MMPI-A Content Scales Assessing Psychopathology in Adolescents.* Minneapolis, MN: University of Minnesota Press.

Chapter 3

ALTERNATIVE EDUCATION PROGRAMS

I N 1991, R. E. MORLEY made the following statement regarding alternative education in a dropout prevention research report:

> Alternative education is a perspective, not a procedure or program. It is based upon the belief that there are many ways to become educated, as well as many types of environments and structures within which this may occur. Further, it recognizes that all people can be educated and that it is in society's interest to ensure that all are educated to at least . . . [a] general high school . . . level. To accomplish this requires that we provide a variety of structures and environments such that each person can find one that is sufficiently comfortable to facilitate progress. (p. 8)

Morley's statement implies two goals that drive the establishment of alternative education programs. The first goal is to help young people become productive members of society. The second goal is the need to remove disruptive influences and to create classrooms that are not only productive, but also safe. In other words, these two goals: (1) the desire to increase graduation rates, and (2) the need to eliminate disruptive or violent students from the classroom without sending them into the streets are viewed as the dual catalysts for policymakers to embrace alternative education.

REACHING THE GOALS

In 1993, the Office of Educational Research and Improvement of the U.S. Department of Education published a booklet entitled *Reaching The Goals, Goal 2: High School Completion*. This booklet, prepared by the Goal 2 Work Group, highlights a variety of individual and family demographic and socioeconomic factors related to dropout rates in the United States. Goal 2 is a policy goal to create school environments that are attractive to dropouts and promote recovery. The Goal 2 Work Group (1993) suggests that a key contribution to the advancement of Goal 2 is the design and support of research that informs educators and the public about the aspects of students' experiences that determine whether or not these students graduate from or complete secondary school. They point out the need to develop and advance theoretical concepts that treat retention, graduation, and completion as consequences of a dynamic interaction of such variables as student characteristics, school context, occupational prospects, and cultural influences.

Researchers have found that dropping out of school is a process. Students do not make snap judgments to leave school. Although the reasons most commonly offered by students for leaving school, such as low grades, inability to get along, working, and pregnancy, are valid, the reasons may not be the true causes but merely rationalizations or simplifications of more complex circumstances. However, dropping out of high school is not an irrevocable action. Notably, approximately two-thirds of dropouts who later complete high school do so by obtaining equivalency credentials such as the General Education Development (GED) credential.

In examining students and their environments, the Goal 2 Work Group (1993) found that individual differences or changes occurring in the lives of students may affect the likelihood of their dropping out or returning to school. Individual student academic performance, motivation and personality, family background, entry into adult work, and family roles are cited as factors that may impact a student's decision to drop out or return to school.

With respect to school influences, the Goal 2 Work Group (1993) highlights research that has identified three key academic and three key nonacademic influences on students that may determine whether they stay in or drop out of school. The three academic influences are: (1) the difficulty of the academic program, (2) a lack of challenging material and low standards, and (3) the view by students that the academic program is simply irrelevant to their lives. The three nonacademic influences suggest that: (1) some students have weak connections to adults and may come to feel that no one in school cares about them, (2) some students may have weak connections to peers in the school and may shift their attention to friends who are already out of school, and (3) some students may have weak connections to the school as an institution and feel powerless and unsure of what is expected of them.

In addressing academic and nonacademic school influences, the Goal 2 Work Group (1993) made the following recommendations:

> School policies and practices may attempt to promote engagement by revising academic standards of the school curriculum, developing students' skills and abilities through school activities, and making academic programs meaningful to the lives of students and relevant to their future. . . . Schools may want to consider adopting policies and practices designed to strengthen students' bonds to school.

Ultimately, the success of any individual program depends upon its features and its goals. Therefore, the most easily recognized aspects of a successful school or program appear to include such features as its culture or climate, organizational structure, curriculum and instruction, and links to other programs and services.

PROGRESSIVE ALTERNATIVE LEARNING ENVIRONMENTS

In 1997, the State Education Department of the University of the State of New York published the *Introductory Guide to Alternative Education.* This guide is designed to provide the basic information required to start and to maintain an alternative education program or school. The guide includes citations and references to Education Law and the Regulations of the Commissioner of Education. The guide (1997) states the purpose of Alternative Education:

> Alternative learning environments provide options for students to enhance their achievement and fulfill their goals and ambitions. Students respond favorable to alternative structures that draw upon their particular skills, abilities and learning styles. Alternative environments often are on the cutting edge of innovative practices and are geared to assist all students in meeting high standards of academic performance. Over 40,000 students are attending alternative education programs/schools operated by local districts or BOCES. An additional 14,000 compulsory school-aged students are receiving educational programming in childcare agencies, detention facilities, county or state jails, and/or divisions for youth facilities. Add these numbers to the approximately 45,000 students reported by school districts and BOCES to be sufficiently behind in their academic pursuits to qualify for enrollment in high school equivalency diploma programs, and the number of students enrolled in some form of alternative education program approaches 100,000 students.

The guide (1997) points out that the most progressive alternative learning environments possess the following characteristics:

Innovation
Achievement of rigorous academic standards and completion of diploma requirements occur because: (a) instructional staff have the knowledge and skills to teach all students; (b) they use innovative curricula with varied teaching methodologies and technology to focus on individual student needs; (c) a learner-centered program is implemented capitalizing on the individual strengths of the students; and (d) smaller class size and individualized instruction accelerates students' progress.

Autonomy
A well-defined, purposeful organization and management structure provides distinction and autonomy from the regular day school and its programs. This is accomplished through the collaborative efforts of staff, students, parents, and the community.

Empowerment
A team approach with student, teacher, family, and community involvement in curriculum matters and policy fosters a climate of shared responsibility and authority.

The guide (1997) also addresses the most frequently asked questions about alternative education. The two most frequently asked questions relative to student population are:
1. Which students should be in alternative education programs?
2. Can students with disabilities attend alternative education programs?

With respect to the question of which students should be in alternative education programs, the guide (1997) points out that a number of programs address the needs of students that have presented behavioral problems or that have functioned poorly in the traditional school setting. Some programs are especially suited for higher achieving students, others programs are for new immigrants, and a number of programs address the instructional needs of pregnant and parenting teens. In addition, some alternative education programs have been established to satisfy the particular learning styles of individual students.

STUDENTS WITH DISABILITIES

With respect to the question of students with disabilities attending alternative education programs, the guide (1997) states:

> Students with disabilities should be enrolled in the least restrictive environment pursuant to a recommendation by the school district's Committee

on Special Education (CSE). If a CSE recommended placement of a student with a disability in an alternative education program, such student would be eligible to attend that program. Such placement must be stated in the student's Individualized Education Plan (IEP). Students attending alternative education programs remain eligible for special education programs and related services to enable them to fully participate. Students who are classified, as needing special education services should be provided appropriate programs as stated in federal and state law and regulations.

Notably, according to the findings of the Goal 2 Work Group (1993) on the dropout rates of traditionally disadvantaged groups, the dropout rates for students with disabilities are almost 20% higher than for students in the general population. Findings show that dropout rates vary widely according to the nature of the disability. For example, among those with disabilities, students who are emotionally disturbed are three times as likely to leave high school by dropping out. The term *Emotional disturbance* is defined in the Regulations of the Commissioner of Education, Part 200 (2000) to mean a condition exhibiting one or more of the following characteristics over a long period of time and to a marked degree that adversely affects a student's educational performance: (a) an inability to learn that cannot be explained by intellectual, sensory, or health factors; (b) an inability to build or maintain satisfactory interpersonal relationships with peers and teachers; (c) inappropriate types of behavior or feelings under normal circumstances; (d) a generally pervasive mood of unhappiness or depression; or (e) a tendency to develop physical symptoms or fears associated with personal or school problems. The term includes schizophrenia. The term does not apply to students who are socially maladjusted, unless it is determined that they have an emotional disturbance.

The Goal 2 Work Group (1993) points out that the indicators that predict the likelihood of dropping out are the same for students with disabilities as for students who have no apparent disabilities. However, as stated previously, although the reasons most commonly offered by students for leaving school, such as low grades, inability to get along, working, and pregnancy, are valid, the reasons may not be the true causes but merely rationalizations or simplifications of more complex circumstances. As reflected in the 20 percent statistical finding, more complex circumstances could be associated with student manifestations of disabilities or mental disorders.

ALTERNATIVE EDUCATION DEPARTMENT:
MONROE #1 BOCES

In July of 1998, the Monroe #1 Board of Cooperative Educational Services (BOCES) in Fairport, NY officially formed the Alternative Education Department. This department took the alternative programs within BOCES and placed them under one administration. David R. Halpern is the principal of the Alternative Education Department. Mr. Halpern is responsible for the administration of the following programs: (1) Future, (2) Alternative Middle School, (3) Phoenix School, (4) Sunset Academy, (5) World of Work, and (6) MOVE (Make Our Vocations Educational). Prior to this merger, the programs were incorporated into other programs and had no identity of their own. The formation of the Alternative Education Department brought together professions with a common goal. This goal is the education of students in an alternative setting.

The traditional middle and high school settings are not suitable for every student. There are some students who need an alternative setting to be successful in their high school academic careers. The Alternative Education Department believes that all students can be successful. Offering these students small class settings, individualized programs, low student-teacher ratios, and crisis intervention contributes to the students' overall success. Many programs within the department also offer individual and/or group counseling. During the 1999–2000 school year, art therapy was introduced and implemented in the following programs: (1) Future, (2) Alternative Middle School, (3) Sunset Academy, and (4) MOVE. A vocational program is also available to every student. In general, the Alternative Education Department works closely with each individual student and his or her home district to provide the best possible program for the student.

The staff also works closely with parents. Ongoing communication between parents and the staff within the department is considered very important. The staff is ready and willing to talk to parents about problems or concerns. There are routine standard communication vehicles for parents: (1) four marking periods during the school year, (2) four mid-marking period updates from the teachers, and (3) immediate notification of any attendance and truancy issues.

The overall goal of the Alternative Education Department is to prepare the students within its programs for life after high school. This life might include college, a trade school, or going right into the working world. The department believes that students must be as ready as possible for living on their own and be able to support themselves. To accomplish this, most high school age students in the department's programs must either take a vocational course, be employed, or commit to a voluntary community service. The student's involvement in either vocation or volunteerism offers him or her the opportunity to be involved in the "adult" world and experience success.

ALTERNATIVE EDUCATION DEPARTMENT: PROGRAM DESCRIPTIONS

Future

The Future program is a self-contained classroom for young women in grades 9–12, who have become mothers at an early age. The program offers young mothers the opportunity to not only complete their education but also to develop skills that will enable them to become employable and begin to support their families.

Entrance Criteria

1. High school age young women.
2. Must be pregnant or parenting.
3. Classified student referrals are accepted.
4. Students with severe emotional disturbances or learning disabilities will be considered on a case by case basis.

Alternative Middle School

The Alternative Middle School program enables students, who are finding little success in their home middle or junior high school, to make personal changes that will enable them to find success in school. The program uses team teaching, cooperative education, project learning, and community service as avenues of learning.

A typical Alternative Middle School student may have issues around: (1) attendance, (2) motivation, (3) organizational skills, and (4) poor self-image or self-esteem as evidenced by depression, poor hygiene, social withdrawal, or not fitting into the mainstream of school.

Entrance Criteria

A student must:
1. Be between 12 and 14 years of age and in grades 6–8.
2. Be no more than two years behind academically.
3. Have average or above average intelligence.
4. Participate with his or her family in an intake.

A student may not:
1. Have a classified disability.
2. Require intensive mental health, drug or alcohol counseling.
3. Have overly aggressive or violent behaviors.

Phoenix School

Adolescents returning to their high school from alcohol and drug treatment must overcome formidable threats to their sobriety and academic success. The Phoenix School program reflects the collaborative efforts of local school districts, chemical dependency treatment agencies, and Monroe #1 BOCES to address the needs of recovering teens. School personnel and treatment professionals join forces at the Phoenix School to provide short-term transitional school placement for recovering teens prior to returning to their home school. A typical Phoenix School student: (1) has at least average intelligence, (2) is working towards high school completion, (3) can be mildly disabled, and (4) must participate in a treatment program including drug screening.

Entrance Criteria

A student must:
1. Be at risk of relapse if he or she remains in or returns to the home school setting.
2. Be in grades 9–12 with a minimum seventh grade reading level.
3. Have demonstrated a period of abstinence.
4. Be committed to remain abstinent.
5. Have recently completed a primary treatment program (outpatient, inpatient or long-term residential).
6. Have a DSM-IV Diagnosis of Substance Dependence.
7. Be amenable to behavior contracting.
8. Have demonstrated an inability to benefit from a lower level of care.

9. Have a Denial Rating Scale of 4 or 5 (to be administered at intake).
10. The student's family or significant other(s) must be willing to actively participate in the student's program and attend a program intake meeting with the student.

Sunset Academy

The Sunset Academy program is designed for students who have not been successful in any high school program and need an afternoon alternative. There are two sections of this program.

Section 1, regular referral, offers individualized instruction, small group instruction, counseling, and integration into vocational programming when needed. This program is held between 2:00–4:00 p.m. at the Alternative High School on the Monroe #1 BOCES Campus.

Section 2 is designed for students who are on long-term suspensions from their home high schools and are referred after a Superintendent's Hearing. These students are involved in the Home and Hospital Tutoring Services prior to referral. This program is held between 2:00–4:00 p.m. in the Foreman Center on the Monroe #1 BOCES Campus.

Entrance Criteria

The student:
1. Must be in grades 9–12.
2. Must be working towards a high school diploma.
3. Must be referred by home school guidance counselor (section 1) or Superintendent's Hearing (section 2).

World of Work

The World of Work program enables students, who are finding little success in their home district's high school, to make personal changes that will enable them to find more success in school. The World of Work program has two sites. One site is located at the Foreman Center on the Monroe #1 BOCES Campus. The other site is located at the Helmer Nature Center in Irondequoit, NY. Both programs are alternatives for high school students having academic, social, or behavioral difficulties in their home schools.

Entrance Criteria

A student must:
1. Be currently enrolled in a 9–12 grade school program.
2. Be referred by their guidance counselor through their district's PPS director.
3. Fit the criteria of a typical student.
4. Participate with his or her family in an intake.

A student may not:
1. Be classified or a severely disabled student.
2. Require intensive mental health, drug or alcohol counseling.
3. Have overly aggressive or violent behaviors.
4. Be involved with criminal activities.

MOVE (Make Our Vocations Educational) *

The MOVE program prepares students, who are still enrolled in school and have decided that they are not motivated to obtain a high school diploma. This program is an alternative to obtaining the regular high school diploma by offering students a High School Equivalency Diploma after the successful completion of the General Education Development (GED) test.

Entrance Criteria

A student must:
1. Be at least 16 years old and under age 21.
2. Have at least one year of high school experience.
3. Have a reading level of 8th grade or higher.
4. Be able to work independently.
5. Participate with his or her family in an intake prior to admission.

*Adapted from *Alternative Education Program Handbook & Calendar, 1999–2000 School Year* by David R. Halpern. Reprinted with permission.

REFERENCES

American Psychiatric Association. (1994). *Diagnostic and Statistical Manual of Mental Disorders* (4th ed.). Washington, DC: American Psychiatric Association.

Butchart, R. E. (1986). Dropout Prevention through Alternative High Schools: A Study of the National Experience. Elmira, NY: Board of Cooperative Educational Services (BOCES).

Halpern, D. R. (1999). *Alternative Education Department Program Handbook & Calendar, 1999–2000 School Year.* Fairport, NY: Monroe #1 Board of Cooperative Educational Services (BOCES).

Jacobs, B. (1994). Recommendations for Alternative Education: Report to the Joint Select Committee to Review the Central Education Agency. Texas Youth Commission.

Kadel, S. (1994). Reengineering High Schools for Student Success. Palatka, FL: Southeast Regional Vision for Education.

Kershaw, C. A., & Blank, M. A. (1993). Student and Educator Perceptions of the Impact of an Alternative School Structure. Atlanta, GA: American Education Research Association.

Korn, C. V. (1991). Alternative American Schools: Ideals in Action. Albany, NY: State University of New York Press.

Morley, R. E. (1991). Alternative Education: Dropout Prevention Research Reports. Clemson, SC: National Dropout Prevention Center.

OERI Goal 2 Work Group. (1993). *Reaching the Goals, Goal 2: High School Completion.* Washington, DC: Office of Educational Research and Improvement, U. S. Department of Education.

Raywid, M. A. (1994a). Focus Schools: A Genre to Consider. New York: ERIC Clearinghouse on Urban Education Institute for Urban and Minority Education.

Rogers, P. C. (1991). At-Risk Programs: Assessment Issues. Long Island, NY: Center For At-Risk Students.

Southwest Educational Development Laboratory (SEDL). (1995). Alternative Learning Environments. *Insights,* Vol. 6.

State Education Department. (1997). *Introductory Guide to Alternative Education.* Albany, NY: University of the State of New York.

State Education Department. (2000). Regulations of the Commissioner of Education, Pursuant to Sections 207, 3214, 4403, 4404 and 4410 of the Education Law, Part 200–Students with Disabilities. Albany, NY: University of the State of New York.

Chapter 4

EMOTIONS AND LEARNING

PHENOMENOLOGY OF EMOTION

AN EMOTION IS A COMPLEX FEELING state with psychic, somatic, and behavioral components. Phenomenology is the aspect of psychopathology that deals with a person's consciously reported experiences. It is also a branch of philosophy that posits that behavior is determined not by an objective external reality, but by a person's subjective perception of that reality. The phenomenology of emotion is discussed in terms of mood and affect.

Mood is a pervasive and subjectively experienced feeling state. Moods are covert. Moods are what people tell you they feel. Affect is the instantaneous, observable expression of emotion. Affects are overt. Affects are what you see people feeling. Table 1 is a glossary of psychopathologic moods and affects.

A *student with a disability* is defined in the Regulations of the Commissioner of Education, PART 200 (2000) as a student who has not attained the age of 21 prior to September 1st and who is entitled to attend public schools pursuant to section 3202 of the Education Law and who, because of mental, physical or emotional reasons, has been identified as having a disability and who requires special services and programs approved by the department. The terms used in this definition include *Emotional disturbance.*

According to the findings of the Goal 2 Work Group (1993) on the dropout rates of traditionally disadvantaged groups, the dropout rate of students with disabilities is almost 20% higher than for students in the general population. The findings show, for example, that among those with disabilities, students who are emotionally disturbed are three times as likely to leave high school by dropping out.

Table 1.
Psychopathologic Moods and Affects

Mood	Description
Anhedonia	Pervasive inability to perceive and experience pleasure in an action and/or event that is normally pleasurable or satisfying for the individual or most individuals.
Apprehensive	Involves worried expectations or anticipation.
Dysphoric	Any unpleasant mood, including irritable, apprehensive, and dysthymic moods.
Dysthymia	Mood of depression or pervasive sadness.
Elevated	More cheerful than normal for the individual, but is not necessarily psychopathological.
Expansive	A lack of restraint in expressing feelings and overvaluation of one's importance.
Euphoric	An exaggerated sense of well being and contentment.
Euthymia	A normal range of mood without dysphoria or elation.
Irritable	A feeling of tension or nervousness; one feels prickly, easily annoyed, provoked to anger, or frustrated.

Affect	Description
Blunted	Individuals who show almost no emotional lability.
Broad	A normal range of affect.
Constricted	Individuals who look dulled, and speak in a monotone.
Flat	Individuals who appear expressionless.
Inappropriate	Clearly discordant with the content of the individual's speech.
Labile	A range of expression in excess of cultural norms, with repeated, rapid, and abrupt shifts of emotion.

PSYCHOBIOLOGY OF EMOTION

In the article, *"How Emotions Affect Learning,"* Robert Sylwester (1994) highlights how new developments in cognitive science are uncovering the mysteries of emotion and how these findings have much to teach about how students do or do not learn. Emotion is important in education because emotion drives attention, which in turn drives learning and memory. Sylwester (1994) explains:

> Recent developments in the cognitive sciences are unlocking the mysteries of how and where our body/brain processes emotion. This unique melding of the biology and psychology of emotion promises to suggest powerful educational applications. . . . Educators should develop a basic understanding of the psychobiology of emotion to enable them to evaluate emerging educational applications.

Cognition is a process that refers to a broad range of mental "behaviors" including awareness, thinking, reasoning, and judgment. In discussing emotion and reason, Sylwester (1994) highlights the fact that emotion can be a more powerful determinant of behavior than the brain's logical/rational processes. Sylwester states:

> Reason may override our emotions, but it rarely changes our real feelings about an issue. Our emotions allow us to bypass conscious deliberation of an issue, and thus to respond quickly based on almost innate general categorizations of incoming information. This may lead to irrational fears and foolish behavior. Often we don't consciously know why we feel as we do about something or someone. Emotion, like color, exists along a continuum, with a wide range of gradations. We can easily identify many discrete emotions through their standard facial and auditory expressions, but the intensity and meaning of the emotion will vary among people and situations. Moreover, emotional context, like color hue, may affect our perception of emotion.

Sylwester (1994) explains that in order to understand the emotional system and its influence on the capacity to learn, two parts of this system must be examined: (1) the peptide hormones that carry emotional information, and (2) the body and brain structures that activate and regulate emotions. The emotional system is primarily located in the brain, endocrine system, and the immune system but it affects all other organs. Scientists now view the brain and the endocrine and immune systems as an integrated biochemical system. An overview of the interrelationship among the brain, the endocrine and immune systems, and behavior may be helpful in understanding Sylwester's concepts.

The Central Nervous System (CNS) consists of the brain and the spinal cord. The spinal cord has two main functions: (1) it is the center for many reflex actions, and (2) it provides a means of communication between the brain and spinal nerves that leave the cord. The largest and uppermost part of the brain is the *cerebrum*. The cerebrum is considered the seat of conscious mental processes. The outer layer of the cerebrum is called the *cerebral cortex*. It is gray in color and contains cell bodies and short fibers. The cerebrum is divided into halves referred to as the right and left *cerebral hemispheres*. Each hemisphere contains four types of superficial lobes: (1) frontal, (2) parietal, (3) temporal, and (4) occipital. Each of the four lobes contains association areas that receive information from the other lobes and integrates this information into higher and more complex levels of consciousness. The *brain stem* is the central core of the brain that links the spinal cord with the cerebral hemispheres. Table 2 highlights the functions of the cerebral lobes.

Consciousness resides only in the cerebrum, the rest of the brain functions below the level of consciousness. The unconscious brain consists of the cerebellum, hypothalamus, thalamus, and medulla oblongata. The *cerebellum*, the second largest part of the brain, is involved in muscle coordination and the maintenance of body equilibrium. The *hypothalamus* is concerned with homeostasis, or the constancy of the internal environment and regulates a variety of functions essential to survival, including temperature and heart rate, as well as thirst, hunger, sex drive, and sleep. The hypothalamus also controls the pituitary gland and thus it serves as a link between the nervous system and the endocrine system. The *thalamus* relays sensory information to the cerebral cortex and translates impulses into conscious sensations. The thalamus is referred to as the "gatekeeper" to the cerebrum because it alerts the cerebrum to only certain sensory input. We are unaware of many of the sensory impulses received by the Central Nervous System (CNS). The *medulla oblongata* regulates vital involuntary processes such as respiration, circulation, heartbeat, and blood pressure.

The Limbic System, which lies beneath the cerebral cortex, involves portions of the conscious and unconscious brain. It is a complex, linked set of structures (including the hippocampus, amygdala, and hypothalamus) considered responsible for emotions. The *hippocampus* is a long sea horse-shaped brain structure involved in emo-

Table 2.
Functions of the Cerebral Lobes

Lobe	Function
Frontal	Motor areas control movements of voluntary skeletal muscles. Association areas carry on higher intellectual processes, such as those required for concentration, planning, complex problem solving, and judging the consequences of behavior.
Parietal	Sensory areas are responsible for the sensations of temperature, touch, pressure, and pain from the skin. Association areas function in the understanding of speech and in using words to express thoughts and feelings.
Temporal	Sensory areas are responsible for hearing and smelling. Association areas are used in the interpretation of sensory experiences and in the memory of visual scenes, music, and other complex sensory patterns.
Occipital	Sensory areas are responsible for vision. Association areas function in combining visual images with other sensory experiences.

Note. From *Human Anatomy and Physiology*, Fifth Edition, by John W. Hole, Jr. Copyright 1990 by Wm. C. Brown Publishers, Dubuque Iowa. Reproduced with permission of The McGraw-Hill Companies.

tion, motivation, learning, and memory. The *amygdala* is an almond-shaped brain structure that plays a role in emotion, particularly aggression. It also serves memory function. Stimulation of different areas of the limbic system can cause the subjective experiences of pleasure and pain.

Along with the Central Nervous System (CNS), the Endocrine System utilizes chemical messengers called *hormones* to coordinate the functioning of body parts. Hormones produced by endocrine glands are secreted directly into the blood stream. All hormones are carried throughout the body by the blood, but each one affects only a specific body part or parts, referred to as target organs. Hormone substances fall into two basic categories: (1) peptides, and (2) steroids.

The Immune System is the body's defense system against disease. Any foreign or potentially dangerous substance (antigen) stimulates the production of specific proteins (antibodies) by the body's white blood cells (lymphocytes) to fight off the invasion.

Sylwester (1994) refers to peptides as the "Molecular Messengers of

Emotion" and highlights how peptides modulate the broad range of pleasure and pain. He explains:

> Peptides travel throughout our body/brain via our neural networks, circulatory system and air passages. They powerfully affect the decisions we make within the continuum of emotionally charged approaching and retreating behaviors. . . . In effect, the shifts in the body/brain levels of these molecules allocate our emotional energy–what we do, when we do it, and how much energy we expend.

Moyers (1992) points out that at the cellular level, peptides synthesized within one cell attach to receptors on the outside of another sparking increased or decreased cellular actions. If this occurs in large populations of cells, it can affect the individual's emotional state. For example, cell division and protein synthesis are both involved in the emotion-charged body changes during adolescence.

Sylwester (1994) cites cortisol and endorphins as two good examples of peptides that can affect students' behavior in the classroom. A stressor is an event that creates a degree of threat by confronting an individual with a demand for change of some kind, or adaptation. Stressors may be mild or catastrophic. When an individual's inability to fend off danger triggers a stress response, or an idiosyncratic reaction to the demand, the adrenal cortex, an endocrine gland, releases cortisol. Cortisol activates important body/brain defensive responses that vary with the nature and severity of the stressor. Stress responses do not differentiate between physical danger and emotional danger. Sylwester (1994) illustrates this point:

> Because most contemporary stress results from emotional problems, these responses are often maladaptive. For example, a 2nd grader refuses to complete an arithmetic assignment. The irritated teacher's stress system inappropriately responds by releasing clotting elements into the blood, elevating cholesterol levels, depressing the immune system, tensing large muscles, increasing the blood pressure–and much more. It's a response that makes sense only if the recalcitrant student is also threatening with a knife or gun.

While low levels of cortisol can produce euphoria, or an exaggerated sense of well being and contentment, high levels of cortisol triggered by the stress response can induce dysphoria, or any unpleasant mood, including irritable, apprehensive, and dysthymic moods. In addition, chronic stress can lead to circulatory, digestive, and immune disorders. It is evident that a high price is paid for chronic emotional stress.

According to Vincent (1990), chronic high cortisol levels can eventually destroy hippocampus neurons, which are involved in emotion, motivation, learning, and memory. Gazzaniga (1989) points out that even short-term stress-related elevation of cortisol in the hippocampus can hinder the ability to distinguish between important and unimportant elements of a memorable event. In essence, stressful school environments significantly reduce the school's ability to carry out its principal mission.

By contrast and more positively, endorphins are called the body's own natural opioids. Endorphins modulate emotions within the pleasure-pain continuum. The opioids are believed to alleviate pain by preventing the release of a neurotransmitter referred to as substance P from certain sensory neurons in the region of the spinal cord. When substance P is released, pain is felt and when substance P is not released, pain is not felt. Evidence also indicates that there are opioid receptors in neurons that travel from the spinal cord to the limbic system and that stimulation of these can cause a feeling of pleasure. Sylwester (1994) explains:

> Endorphin levels can be elevated by exercise and by positive social contacts (hugging, music, a friend's supportive comments, among other things), thereby making us feel good about ourselves and our social environment. A joyful classroom atmosphere that encourages such behaviors produces internal chemical responses in students that make them more apt to learn how to successfully solve problems in potentially stressful situations.

In essence, the endorphins contribute to adaptive behavior, or the effectiveness with which the individual copes with the natural and social demands of the environment. The ability to cope suggests the capacity to manage emotionally arousing situations.

The endocrine and immune systems participate in the processing of emotions. The interrelated brain systems that share the task of regulating the emotions are the brain stem, limbic system, and cerebral cortex. According to Vincent (1990), extensively connected in looped circuits to body organs and systems, the brain stem and limbic system responds slowly (from seconds to months) as it regulates basic body functions, cycles, and defenses. The system has a large quantity of peptide receptors. The *reticular activating system*, sometimes referred to as the reticular formation, located at the top of the brain stem, integrates the amount and type of incoming sensory information into a general level of attention.

As previously stated, the thalamus is a central relay station for sensory impulses traveling upward from other parts of the spinal cord and the brain to the cerebrum. It receives all sensory impulses and channels them to appropriate regions of the cerebrum. The thalamus has connections to various parts of the brain by way of nerve fibers that radiate from the upper part of the reticular activating system. This system, which extends from the medulla to the thalamus, sorts out stimuli received from sense organs including the eyes and ears, passing on only those stimuli that require immediate attention.

In discussing the limbic system and its role in emotion and memory, Sylwester (1994) explains:

> The limbic system, composed of several small, interconnected structures, is our brain's principal regulator of emotion and plays important roles in processing memory. This may explain why emotion is an important ingredient in many memories. The limbic system is powerful enough to override both rational thought and innate brain stem response patterns. In short, we tend to follow our feelings. Memories formed during a specific emotional state tend to be easily recalled during a similar emotional state later. For example, during an argument, we easily recall similar previous arguments. Thus, classroom simulations and role-playing activities enhance learning because they tie memories to the kinds of emotional contexts in which they will later be used.

LEARNING AND MEMORY

Learning requires memory. Basic memory processes include the most fundamental aspects of remembering things: (1) the routine acts of storing information, and (2) retrieving information. Sensory information (environmental input) first enters the sensory registers where it is briefly stored (less than 1 second). Then, whatever information is consciously noted is moved to short-term memory, which is of a more limited capacity but holds information longer (up to 1 minute). Some of the information in short-term memory is moved to long-term memory, which has a very large capacity and holds information for a very long time. Increases in memory capacity and efficiency have both been used to explain cognitive development. It is believed for both types of memory, short-term and long-term, impulses move within the limbic circuit but eventually long-term memories are stored in sensory areas. The involvement of the limbic system explains why emotionally charged events result in the most vivid memories and why sensory stimulation can awaken a complex memory.

Information-Processing Model

Note. Adapted from *Child Development: Its Nature and Course*, Second Edition, by L. A. Sroufe, R. G. Cooper, and G. B. DeHart. Copyright 1992 by McGraw-Hill, Inc., New York, NY. Reproduced with permission of The McGraw-Hill Companies.

Piaget (1973) referred to knowledge as memory in the wider sense. Knowledge has a tremendous affect on what individuals are able to learn and remember. The research on the knowledge component of memory has involved constructive memory, which is defined as the recall of new information that is only partly the product of the actual new information just received. Recall of new information is also the product of inferences made on the bases of data previously stored in memory. In other words, what we know influences what we can learn and the ease with which we can assimilate new information.

EMOTION AND MEMORY

Sylwester (1994) discusses the four limbic system structures that process emotion and memory: (1) amygdala, (2) hippocampus, (3) thalamus, and (4) hypothalamus. He states:

• Amygdala Complex. This is the principal limbic system structure involved in processing the emotional content of behavior and memory. It is composed of two small almond-shaped structures that connect our sensory-

motor systems and autonomic nervous system (which regulates such survival functions as breathing and circulation). The amygdala is also richly
and reciprocally connected to most other brain areas. Its principal task is
to filter and interpret sophisticated incoming sensory information in the
context of our survival and emotional needs, and then help initiate appropriate responses. Thus, it influences both early sensory processing and
higher levels of cognition.

• Hippocampus. The amygdala adjoins the hippocampus that converts
  important short-term experiences into long-term declarative memories
  that are stored in the cortex. Think of the amygdala as processing the subjective feelings you associate with an event, and the hippocampus as processing the objective location, time, and actions that defined the event. The
  brain's amygdala and the adjoining hippocampus can modulate the subjective and objective strength of a memory.

• Thalamus. The thalamus informs the rest of our brain about what's happening outside our body. The thalamus has direct connections to the
  amygdala, which permits it to send a very rapid but factually limited report
  on a potential threat. This can trigger a quick, emotionally loaded (perhaps
  life-saving) behavior before we fully understand what's happening. And it
  is the mechanism that underlies many explosive outbursts during a typical
  school day.

• Hypothalamus. The hypothalamus monitors our internal regulatory systems, informing our brain what's happening inside our body. When our
  brain has no solution to a threatening situation, the hypothalamus can activate a fight-flight stress response through its pituitary gland contacts with
  the endocrine gland system.

Slywester (1994) describes the cerebral cortex as a large sheet of
neural tissue that is "deeply folded around the limbic system." The
cerebral cortex: (1) receives, categorizes, and interprets sensory information, (2) makes rational decisions, and (3) activates behavioral
responses. In discussing the functions of the right and left cerebral
hemispheres, Sylwester points out:

> Although the research isn't conclusive on the roles the hemispheres (or
> lobes) play in emotion, some general patterns are apparent. The right hemi-
> sphere seems to play the more prominent role overall in processing emo-
> tions. It processes the important emotional content of faces, gestures, and
> language (intonation, volume)–how something was communicated; while
> the left hemisphere processes much of the objective content of language–
> what was said. The right hemisphere processes the negative aspects that lead
> to withdrawal behaviors (for example, fear and disgust), while the left hemi-
> sphere processes the positive aspects of emotion that lead to approaching
> behaviors (for example, laughter and joy).

IMPLICATIONS OF EMOTION RESEARCH

Sylwester (1994) explains that although the educational applications of emotion research are still tentative, several general themes have emerged. He identifies these general principles and their applications to the classroom:

1. We should seek to develop forms of self-control among students and staff that encourages nonjudgmental, nondisruptive . . . venting of emotion.
2. Schools should focus more on metacognitive activities that encourage students to talk about their emotions, listen to their classmates' feelings, and think about the motivations of people who enter their curricular world. Metacognition greatly increases the ability to plan effective problem-solving strategies. For example, the simple use of why in a question turns the discussion away from bare facts and toward motivations and emotions.
3. Activities that emphasize social interaction and that engage the entire body tends to provide the most emotional support. Games, discussions, field trips, interactive projects, cooperative learning, physical education, and the arts are examples.
4. Memories are contextual. School activities that draw out emotions (simulations, role playing, and cooperative projects, for example) may provide important contextual memory prompts that will help students recall the information during closely-related events in the real world.
5. Emotionally stressful school environments are counterproductive because they can reduce students' ability to learn. Self-esteem and a sense of control over one's environment are important in managing stress.

With respect to how emotions affect learning, it may be helpful to review the definition of *Emotional disturbance* as defined in the Regulations of the Commissioner of Education, PART 200 (2000). The term *Emotional disturbance* means a condition exhibiting one or more of the following characteristics over a long period of time and to a marked degree that adversely affects a student's educational performance: (a) an inability to learn that cannot be explained by intellectual, sensory, or health factors; (b) an inability to build or maintain satisfactory interpersonal relationships with peers and teachers; (c) inappropriate types of behavior or feelings under normal circumstances; (d) a generally pervasive mood of unhappiness or depression; or (e) a tendency to develop physical symptoms or fears associated with personal or school problems. The term includes schizophrenia. The term does not apply to students who are socially maladjusted, unless it is determined that they have an emotional disturbance.

Etiology refers to the origins of a disorder. Advances in psychobiology and epidemiology, which is the science that studies the frequency and distribution of disorders within various populations, have both contributed to a better understanding of etiology. When exploring the dimensions of "causation," formulations must consider the diverse etiological influences such as initiation, perpetuation, exacerbation, and predisposition. What initiates a disorder usually differs from what perpetuates it. What originates and maintains a problem may also differ from what exacerbates a disorder. A predisposition, or a latent susceptibility to a disorder, may be activated under certain conditions such as stress.

At the beginning of the twentieth century, education reformers made eloquent pleas for the education of the "whole" child. As evidenced through the advances in the psychobiology of emotion, a student must be thought of as more than brain tissue and body. Powerful hormones are converting body and brain tissue into a vibrant life force, fashioning not only the mental and physical components but also the social and emotional components, which encompass the "whole" child that must be educated in the twenty-first century.

REFERENCES

Chaplin, J. P. (1985). *Dictionary of Psychology* (2nd Revised Edition). New York: Dell Publishing Co., Inc.

Gazzaniga, M. (1989). *Mind Matters: How Mind and Brain Interact to Create Our Conscious Lives.* Boston, MA: Houghton Mifflin.

Hole, J. W., Jr. (1990). *Human Anatomy and Physiology* (5th ed.). Dubuque, IA: Wm. C. Brown Publishers.

Kaplan, H. I., & Sadock, B. J. (1991). *Comprehensive Glossary of Psychiatry and Psychology.* Baltimore, MD: Williams & Wilkins.

Mader, S. S. (1992). *Human Biology* (3rd ed.). Dubuque, IA: Wm. C. Brown Publishers.

Maxmen, J. S., & Ward, N. G. (1995). *Essential Psychopathology and Its Treatment* (2nd edition Revised for DSM-IV). New York: W. W. Norton & Company.

Moyers, B. (1992). *Healing and the Mind.* New York: Doubleday.

OERI Goal 2 Work Group. (1993). *Reaching the Goals, Goal 2: High School Completion.* Washington, DC: Office of Educational Research and Improvement, U. S. Department of Education.

Piaget, J., & Inhelder, B. (1973). *Memory and Intelligence.* New York: Basic Books.

Restak, R. M. (1988). *The Mind.* New York: Bantam Books.

Shirk, S. R. (Ed.). (1988). *Cognitive Development and Child Psychotherapy.* New York: Plenum Press.

Sroufe, L. A., Cooper, R. G., & DeHart, G. B. (1992). *Child Development: Its Nature and Course* (2nd ed.). New York: McGraw-Hill, Inc.

Statt, D. (1981). *Dictionary of Psychology*. New York: Harper & Row, Publishers.

State Education Department. (2000). Regulations of the Commissioner of Education, Pursuant to Sections 207, 3214, 4403, 4404 and 4410 of the Education Law, PART 2000 – Students with Disabilities. Albany, NY: University of the State of New York.

Sylwester, R. (1994). How Emotions Affect Learning. *Educational Leadership*, Vol. 52, No. 2, 60–65.

Vincent, J.D. (1990). The Biology of Emotions. Cambridge, MA: Basil Blackwell.

Chapter 5

ART THERAPY IN THE SCHOOLS

SCHOOL ART THERAPY:
IMPLICATIONS FOR FUTURE CHANGE

IN THE ARTICLE, "*The Development of School Art Therapy in Dade County Public Schools: Implications for Future Change,*" Janet Bush (1997) highlights the variety of tasks that must be accomplished to make art therapy an integral part of the educational program and how it will accommodate changing times.

During the 1979–1980 school year, the Dade County, Miami, Florida public school system began providing art therapy treatment for students with physical, emotional, educational, and psychological problems. Bush (1997) points out that the initial purpose of implementing the program was to, "ameliorate a variety of unacceptable behaviors and to help the students learn by improvement of the students' insight, attitudes, and skills." She highlights the fact that in a school setting, art therapists are not only qualified to observe and analyze behavior, art products, and students' communications, but also to make diagnostic assessments based on the students' art products and to formulate treatment plans.

Bush (1997) explains:

> Art therapists utilize art and individual association with art products to help generate physical, emotional, and learning skills that foster compatible relationships between the students and their inner and outer worlds. Students who are helped through art therapy to come to an improved understanding of their problems are often able to follow through and resolve their problems.

Bush (1997) points out that today's students are challenged by a variety of concerns that can directly and indirectly affect their educational progress and that by means of art products, art therapists are able to assist the students in meeting and resolving their problems. Art therapists can provide individual counseling, group procedures, consultations with parents and teachers, and referrals to the appropriate agencies and professionals in the community. She stresses that the focus is on developmental issues and addressing critical concerns that pose an immediate threat to the individual student's social, emotional, and psychological well being.

PUBLIC LAW 94-142 AND PUBLIC LAW 105-17

The Education for All Handicapped Children Act of 1975, Public Law 94-142, in its original form, identified art therapy as a viable service that might benefit a child who required special education. Public Law 94-142 made it possible for school systems to allocate monies to help fund art therapy. The Individuals with Disabilities Education Act Amendments of 1997, Public Law 105-17, strengthens academic expectations and accountability for the nation's 5.8 million children with disabilities. The classification of disabilities include: mental retardation, hearing impairment (including deafness), speech or language impairment, visual impairment (including blindness), emotional disturbance, orthopedic impairment, autism, traumatic brain injury, other health impairment, or specific learning disabilities.

POSITION PAPER OF THE AMERICAN ART THERAPY ASSOCIATION

Bush (1997) references the 1985 monograph published by the American Art Therapy Association (AATA) entitled, "*Art Therapy in the Schools: A Position Paper of the American Art Therapy Association.*" The monograph includes a *Resource Packet for Art Therapists in Schools.* The monograph is intended for individuals and groups responsible for school art therapy programs in the United States—art therapists, school board members, administrators, and others who might be concerned with the application of art therapy in the schools. Bush (1997) states, "It reflected the official position of the American Art Therapy Association, which was directed toward the promotion and recognition of educationally sound art therapy programs in the U.S." The position paper and resource packet provide a foundation for current work promoting school art therapy.

The *Resource Packet for Art Therapists in Schools* (1985) includes the following:
- Sample Job Descriptions for an Art Therapist
- Sample Art Therapy Job Specifications
- Regulations and Procedures for Public Law 94-142
- Identifying Art Therapy Candidates
- Referral Form for Diagnostic Art Therapy Assessment
- Annotated Bibliography of Diagnostic Art Therapy Procedures for Children and Adolescents
- Confidentiality and Release Forms for Use in Art Therapy
- Art Therapy Goals and Short Term Objectives
- Model Art Therapy Progress Notes Form
- Guidelines for Using Art Therapy Intake Record
- Supplies and Materials for Art Therapy

In introducing the resource packet, AATA (1985) points out:

> For those art therapists who work in a program governed by P.L. 94-142, this publication should prove to be a worthwhile resource. For those art therapists who work in educational settings not influenced by this public law, this resource packet should undoubtedly provide reference material of use to any art therapy program. The material may be adapted to suit the needs of art therapists working under state department of public instruction rules and regulations, and a particular school district's educational policy.

TARGET POPULATIONS

In discussing target populations in the monograph, AATA (1985) expanded the population scope to include children who are not identified as disabled, but who may experience difficulty in school as a result of social or emotional problems. AATA (1985) discusses this broader view of school art therapy:

> Art therapy assists them in achieving an appropriate level of social and academic performance. Difficulties associated with nonschool environments may be related to a crisis in the home, such as the death of a significant person, parental separation or divorce, physical or mental ailments, physical or psychological abuse, and other disruptive circumstances. The supportive service and direct involvement of an art therapist in the school can help to address, assess, and remediate those specific issues. Behavior problems not visible at home but exhibited at school may be caused by academic-related difficulties, transferring to a new school, peer pressure, problems in socialization, and difficulty with authority figures. The resolution of conflicts during a child's educational career may result in more successful school adjust-

ment and more productive adult experiences. Art therapy is applicable to, and appropriate for, students at all age levels, from preschool through senior high school and it offers a therapeutic diagnostic and prescriptive approach. Continued efforts should be made to strengthen the program for those students identified as handicapped, and also to develop programs for students who, although not identified as handicapped, would profit from the art therapy treatment.

CREATING A SUCCESSFUL PARTNERSHIP:
ART THERAPY AND PUBLIC SCHOOLS

In highlighting the pilot program in the Dade County Public Schools, Bush (1997) explains that the initial program combined both art education objectives and art therapy objectives for selected disabled students in self-contained classrooms. As programs for the severely emotionally disturbed students increased, and as the services of art therapists were expanded, the art education component was eliminated from the schedule of the art therapists. Bush (1997) explains:

> This provided the art therapist with more time to (1) implement clinical art therapy objectives, (2) see more individual students and small groups of students, (3) do further assessment and diagnostic work-ups, and (4) meet with parents and treatment team personnel to collaborate on student cases. This revised approach was developed to provide treatment for troubled children, not to impart curriculum art objectives. It concentrated on art as psychotherapy, leaving the application of cultural art goals to the art education teachers who were a normal complement of the school program.

Currently the art therapy program has 21 full-time art therapists who are staff members of the Dade County Public Schools Division of Exceptional Student Education. Each therapist is assigned to a site serving severely emotionally disturbed students. The title "Clinical Art Therapy Department" is used to emphasize the distinction between art therapy and the fields of art education and psychology.

Bush (1997) raises the question, "Will art therapy eventually be well established in all school systems, and will it serve as one accepted means of addressing student failure in the classroom?" She answers by stating that it depends on a growing appreciation of the merits of art therapy. Bush notes that there are gaps that exist in the efforts to establish the notion that art therapy belongs in the schools. She identifies major issues and suggests ways that these should be addressed:

1. State Certification / Credentialing Action:
   If school art therapy is to grow, art therapists will need to work toward meeting individual state requirements for licensure or certification.
2. Graduate Level Preparation to Meet the Needs of Practitioners:
   Graduate students need to be given the opportunity to specialize in school art therapy and to be able to acquire a body of knowledge that will prepare them to introduce and implement effective school art therapy programs.
3. National Guidelines for Comprehensive School Art Therapy Programs:
   The schools have always considered psychotherapy a private endeavor best left outside the school. In today's climate, teachers, administrators, and parents must be helped to understand their biases and the benefits that may be obtained by recognizing the relationship between learning and mental health. Art therapists must become proactive in defining the contribution that art therapy makes to learning.
4. Funding for School Art Therapy:
   A basic budget for a program includes expenditures such as personnel costs for full-time or part-time therapists as well as money for art supplies. Individual art therapists may be the persons best able to educate administrators to the benefits inherent in an art therapy approach and to persuade districts to budget for art therapy expenses.
5. Developing a Role and Purpose for Art Therapy in Schools:
   What is needed is an understanding that school art therapists are highly trained professionals who offer specific skills and services to help students with their educational and emotional development. This is the primary role of the art therapist in schools. They are different from art therapists who practice in clinics, hospitals, and other setting, but this difference is simply a reflection of the educational and developmental focus of their programs and services.
6. The Absence of Documentation and Research on School Art Therapy:
   The time has come for art therapists working in school environments to produce and disseminate documentation that will educate consumers and school personnel to art therapy's potential.
7. The Promoting and Marketing of School Art Therapy by Art Therapists:
   An art therapist must be an advocate, promoter, and ambassador for the schools; this means communicating with everyone.

Bush (1997) cautions that the future of school art therapy as a profession will depend on the ability of art therapists to become an important and integral part of the school setting. They must maintain their unique role while contributing to the learning process. She advocates that art therapy and public school education can be a successful partnership. Together they can provide the tools with which to lead students to self-expression and ultimately into cognitive, emotional, and social growth.

REFERENCES

American Art Therapy Association. (1985). *Art Therapy in the Schools: A Position Paper of the American Art Therapy Association.* Mundelein, IL: American Art Therapy Association, Inc.

American Art Therapy Association. (1985). *Resource Packet for Art Therapists in Schools.* Mundelein, IL: American Art Therapy Association, Inc.

Arena, J. (1978). *How to Write an I.E.P.* Novato, CA: Academic Therapy Publications.

Ballard, J., Ramierez, B., & Zantal-Wiener, K. (1987). Public Law 94-142, Section 504 And Public Law 99-457: Understanding What They Are and Are Not. Reston, VA: The Council for Exceptional Children.

Bush, J. (1997). The Development of School Art Therapy in Dade County Public Schools: Implications for Future Change. *Journal of the American Art Therapy Association,* Vol. 14, 9–14.

Bush, J. (1997). *The Handbook of School Art Therapy: Introducing Art Therapy into a School System.* Springfield, IL: Charles C Thomas.

Education for All Handicapped Children Act of 1975, Public Law 94-142, (1975).

Individuals with Disabilities Education Act of 1990, Public Law 101-476, (1990).

Individuals with Disabilities Education Act Amendments of 1997, Public Law 105-17, (1997).

State Education Department. (2000). Regulations of the Commissioner of Education, Pursuant to Sections 207, 3214, 4403, 4404 and 4410 of the Education Law, PART 200 – Students with Disabilities. Albany, NY: University of the State of New York.

Chapter 6

IMPLEMENTATION OF THE
ART THERAPY PROGRAM

RATIONALE FOR THERAPEUTIC INTERVENTION

A BRIDGE IS A STRUCTURE spanning and providing passage over an obstacle. As a metaphor, the concept of a bridge may be applied to adolescence. Adolescence is the bridge that spans the developmental period between childhood and adulthood. This developmental period is filled with cognitive, social, and emotional challenges.

In addition to the normal developmental challenges, the adolescents referred to the Alternative Education Department at Monroe #1 BOCES are considered to be "at risk." This term, within the educational system, refers to students with the potential for displaying academic, behavioral, and social problems. Academically at-risk students fail to achieve and are predictably dropout prone. Behaviorally at-risk students display inappropriate school behaviors. Socially at-risk students are faced with school disciplinary charges and may have been brought to the attention of the juvenile justice system. As research has pointed out, the desire to increase graduation rates and the need to eliminate disruptive or violent students from the classroom without sending them into the streets are viewed as the dual catalysts for policymakers to embrace alternative education.

Researchers also suggest that the professionals designing alternative education programs should consider both the at-risk factors and the personality characteristics of alternative education students in order to develop effective interventions. Six factors have been isolated that describe the attitudes and personality characteristics of these students: (1) defensiveness/hopelessness, (2) attention seeking, (3) antisocial disorders, (4) conduct disorders, (5) interpersonal problems, and (6) family relationship problems. The recommendations made by

Fuller and Sabatino (1996) are restated because they underscore the need for effective interventions:

> Given the personality characteristics of this group, the need for individual psychological assessment of each student entering an alternative program becomes apparent. Many students currently placed in alternative school programs would qualify for special education services following psychological evaluation. Some would be learning disabled, some seriously emotionally disturbed, and some comorbid with both conditions. To be effective, alternative school programs should include intensive individual and group counseling focusing on self-esteem, self-concept, personality, responsibility, appropriate expression of feelings, drug/alcohol prevention, vocational assessment, and career exploration and preparation. Family counseling could be an integral phase of treatment if the participation of parents/caregivers is obtained. These students must be convinced of their own self-worth and be able to foresee the consequences of the choices they make.

The developmental challenges of adolescence coupled with the at-risk factors and the attitudes and personality characteristics of alternative education students underscore the need for counseling. Therefore, an individual and/or group experience can provide the opportunity for these students to explore issues and problems and to find ways of making responsible choices.

Marianne Schneider Corey and Gerald Corey (1997) highlight the suitability of group counseling for adolescents:

> Group counseling is especially suitable because adolescents can identify and experience their conflicting feelings, discover that they're not unique in their struggles, openly question those values they decide to modify, learn to communicate with peers and adults, learn from the modeling provided by the leader, and learn how to accept what others offer and to give of themselves in return. Adolescents often need to learn to label and verbalize their feelings. Groups provide a place where they can safely experiment with reality and test their limits. A unique value of group counseling is that it lets adolescents be instrumental in one another's growth; group members help one another in the struggle for self-understanding. Most important, a group gives adolescents a chance to express themselves and to be heard and to interact with their peers. (pp. 324–325)

ART THERAPY

Definition of the Profession

The profession of Art Therapy is defined by the American Art

Therapy Association (1990) as:

> A human service profession that utilizes art media, images, the creative process, and patient/client responses to the created products as reflections of an individual's development, abilities, personality, interests, concerns, and conflicts. Art therapy practice is based on the knowledge of human development and psychological theories, which are implemented in a full spectrum of models of assessment and treatment including educational, psychodynamic, cognitive, transpersonal, and other therapeutic means of reconciling emotional conflicts, fostering self-awareness, developing social skills, managing behavior, solving problems, reducing anxiety, aiding reality orientation, and increasing self-esteem.

Titles and Scope of Practice

In 1997, the American Art Therapy Association (AATA) disseminated a Title and Scope of Practice. A professional art therapist has completed the requirements for professional membership set forth by the American Art Therapy Association (AATA). These requirements include the successful completion of a graduate art therapy educational program and supervised art therapy practicum. A registered art therapist has successfully completed the requirements for Art Therapist Registered (ATR) set forth by the Art Therapy Credentials Board (ATCB). A board certified art therapist has completed the requirements for Art Therapist Registered (ATR) and has passed a certificate examination administered by the Art Therapy Credentials Board (ATCB).

Ethical Standards

An ethic is a principle of right or good conduct or a body of such principles. Ethical codes constitute the rules professional members must adhere to in their practices. In 2001, the American Art Therapy Association (AATA) disseminated an Ethics Document to its members. The Statement of Purpose in the document reads:

> The purpose of this ethics document is to define and establish ethical behavior for current and future members of this association, and to inform credentialing bodies, employers of art therapists, and the general public that members of the American Art Therapy Association, Inc. are required to adhere to the *Ethical Standard for Art Therapists.* This document includes procedures for handling complaints of violations of these standards.

Members of the American Art Therapy Association must abide by these standards and by applicable state laws and regulations governing the conduct of art therapists and any additional license or certification, which the art therapist holds. The Ethical Standards for Art Therapists* (2001) include the following:

1.0 RESPONSIBILITY TO CLIENTS
Art therapists shall advance the welfare of all clients, respect the rights of those persons seeking their assistance, and make reasonable efforts to ensure that their services are used appropriately.

2.0 CONFIDENTIALITY
Art therapists shall respect and protect confidential information obtained from clients in conversation and/or through artistic expression.

3.0 ASSESSMENT METHODS
Art therapists develop and use assessment methods to better understand and serve the needs of their clients. They use assessment methods only within the context of a defined professional relationship.

4.0 PUBLIC USE AND REPRODUCTION OF CLIENT ART EXPRESSION AND THERAPY SESSIONS
Art therapists shall not make or permit any public use or reproduction of the clients' art therapy sessions, including dialogue and art expression, without express written consent of the client.

5.0 PROFESSIONAL COMPETENCE AND INTEGRITY
Art therapists shall maintain high standards of professional competence and integrity.

6.0 MULTICULTURAL COMPETENCE
Cultural competence is a set of congruent behaviors, attitudes, and policies that enable art therapists to work effectively in cross-cultural situations. Art therapists acknowledge and incorporate into their professional work the importance of culture; variations within cultures; the assessment of cross-cultural relations; cultural differences in visual symbols and imagery; vigilance towards the dynamics that result from cultural differences; the expansion of cultural knowledge; and the adaptation of services to meet culturally-unique needs.

7.0 RESPONSIBILITY TO STUDENTS AND SUPERVISEES
Art therapists shall instruct their students using accurate, current, and scholarly information and will, at all times, foster the professional growth of students and advisees.

8.0 RESPONSIBILITY TO RESEARCH PARTICIPANTS
Researchers shall respect the dignity and protect the welfare of participants in research.

9.0 RESPONSIBILITY TO THE PROFESSION
Art therapists shall respect the rights and responsibilities of colleagues and participate in activities which advance the goals of art therapy.

ART THERAPY IN AN EDUCATIONAL ENVIRONMENT

The 1985 monograph published by the American Art Therapy Association (AATA) entitled, "*Art Therapy in the Schools: A Position Paper of the American Art Therapy Association,*" provides information and guidelines designed to establish a foundational framework for implementing a sound art therapy program in an educational environment. Table 3 is a sample job description for an art therapist working in an educational setting. The American Art Therapy Association (1985) provides a working definition of art therapy in the schools:

> Art therapy is a psychoeducational therapeutic intervention that focuses upon art media as primary expressive and communicative channels. The art therapy process allows one to explore personal problems and potentials through nonverbal and verbal expression and to develop physical, emotional and/or learning skills through therapeutic art experiences. In art therapy the child can directly manipulate materials and the environment, symbolically exploring, organizing and assimilating meaning from a complex world of ideas and experiences. This process may facilitate order, reduce confusion and uncertainty, and promote the integration of experiences. This integrative process is important for children as they experience, communicate, and negotiate through developmental levels . . . . Art therapy can facilitate appropriate social behavior and promote healthy affective development so that children can become more receptive to learning, realizing their social and academic potential. Therefore, art therapy in a school, whether public or private, can be relevant to a child's education and social and emotional maturation.

Harriet Wadeson (1980) identifies certain unique advantages that art expression contributes to therapeutic interventions. These advantages include:

• *Imagery.* Images form the base of experience in personality development. We think in images. Images are also the primary component of unconscious phenomena for reflection. Art media can stimulate the production of images.

• *Decreased Defenses.* Since art is a less customary communication vehicle for most individuals, it is less amenable to control. Unexpected depictions or symbols may appear in a drawing, painting, or sculpture that are contrary to the intentions of the creator. These can lead to unexpected recognition, which in turn can enhance insight and promote learning and growth.

• *Objectification.* The art expression can form a bridge. This process is referred to as objectification because thoughts and feelings are at first

Table 3.
Job Description for an Art Therapist in an Educational Setting

---

Position: Art Therapist

Qualifications: Master's degree (or equivalent) in art therapy from an accredited
                   program in art therapy OR professionally registered by the American
                   Art Therapy Association (AATA).

Responsibilities and Duties:
• Plan, organize, and develop an art therapy program designed to meet the individually
  assessed special needs of children ages 0-21.
• Establish criteria for referral to art therapy and eligibility of each candidate.
• Administer diagnostic art therapy evaluations to referred students to determine eligibility
  for services.
• Develop individualized appropriate goals and objectives for students, based upon informa-
  tion concerning the student's emotional, perceptual, cognitive, physical, and social level of
  functioning gleaned from the art therapy diagnostic procedure and student's case history.
• Document interpretations of the evaluation and recommendations for treatment in a narra-
  tive report including individualized goals and objectives.
• Incorporate the student's art therapy goals and objectives into an Individualized Education
  Program (IEP).
• Implement treatment plan by providing individual and/or group services as specified by
  the IEP.
• Reevaluate students at appropriate intervals, changing treatment plan as indicated.
• Assess and document effectiveness of treatment plan for the student, citing strategies and
  techniques used in striving toward specified objectives in a narrative report, at least on an
  annual basis.
• Participate in ongoing staff meetings with interdisciplinary treatment team, collaborating
  with significant participants involved in case management.
• Communicate progress and results of art therapy services to educational staff, related service providers, parents, and when appropriate and approved, to other professionals treat-
  ing the student.
• Participate in IEP conferences.
• Conduct in-service lectures, workshops, and presentations and participate in staff develop-
  ment activities for personnel.
• Perform administrative tasks such as maintaining records, materials, and equipment, requi-
  sitioning of supplies, and organizing the art therapy room.
• Maintain case histories including descriptions or slides of artwork and interpretation thereof.
• Continue educational endeavors and continue professional competency.
• Engage in individual or collaborative art therapy research.
• Supervise art therapy interns as indicated.
• Assist in all other departmental activities and duties as indicated.

---

externalized in the art object. The art object allows the individual to recognize the existence of these thoughts and feelings and if owned by the individual, may become integrated as part of the self.

- *Permanence.* The drawing, painting, or sculpture is not subject to the distortions of memory. It remains the same and can be recalled intact over an extended period of time after its creation.
- *Spatial Matrix.* Verbalization is linear communication. Art expression is spatial. There is no time element. In art expression, relationships occur in space not time.
- *Creative and Physical Energy.* Art can become a way of knowing and learning about the self through the processes inherent in drawing, painting, and sculpture.

ART THERAPY GOALS AND OBJECTIVES

The goals and objectives identified for the Alternative Education Department at Monroe #1 BOCES were developed based upon the guidelines established by the American Art Therapy Association (1985). Table 4 highlights the goals and measurable objectives for: (1) cognitive growth, (2) emotional regulation, and (3) social behavior.

DIAGNOSTIC ASSESSMENT

Assessment is the process of gathering evidence in order to make some informed judgment. It is a specific task distinct from therapy. Within an educational environment, the art therapist is advised to administer a diagnostic art therapy assessment to ascertain the cognitive and emotional development of the student. Janet Bush (1997) points out:

> An assessment can help to determine the appropriateness of student placement in art therapy as well as provide base line data on the student, and serve to establish goals and objectives for treatment. The assessment may be implemented prior to placement in a special program, in conjunction with the psychological testing process, or it may be used after the youngster has been placed in a special program to provide further information about the youngster. Schools are advised to implement the procedures that would be most beneficial to their programming needs. (p. 51)

The procedures implemented for identifying and referring students in the Alternative Education Department at Monroe #1 BOCES for a

Table 4.
Alternative Education Department / Monroe #1 BOCES
Art Therapy Goals and Objectives

Cognitive Growth	Emotional Regulation	Social Behavior
Goal: Through the process of art therapy, the student will demonstrate improved skills in cognitive functioning.	Goal: Through the process of art therapy, the student will develop recognition of, and consequently a better regulation of emotional drives. The student will develop a self-image based on feelings of competency and adequacy through participation in art therapy group and/or individual sessions.	Goal: Through the process of art therapy, the student will experiment with a broader repertoire of adaptive interpersonal behaviors.
Objectives: Expression of Thought: The student will organize intellectual concepts in graphic form during 75% of the time. Flexibility: The student will demonstrate skills in spontaneity yet inhibit impulsiveness 50% of the time. Attending/Focusing: The student will use art as a means of focusing thoughts and carry through with ideas in a logical, sequential progression 75% of the time. Communication: The student will improve graphic expression of thoughts and feelings and promote a depth of self-expression via art by 50% of his/her present level.	Objectives: Self-Monitoring / Evaluating: The student will develop skills in reflective approaches to his/her artwork measured by 50% improvement over his/her present level of functioning. Control: The student will strengthen control over cognitive associative functioning as indicated in graphic representation. Reality Testing / Sublimation: The student will use art as a means of testing and verifying reality ties during 80% of the opportunities given. The student will sublimate sexual and aggressive impulses into more appropriate and acceptable channels during 80% of opportunities given. Release of Emotions: The student will reconcile feelings of anger (or stress, frustration, vulnerability, dependency needs, etc.) via creating art in an art therapy setting. Self Image: The student will attempt self-confrontation in terms of feelings related to self-image and concept during 50% of the opportunities given.	Objectives: Maturation: The student will develop and demonstrate a more mature posture during 80% of the opportunities given as measured by the student's behavior, verbalizations, and works of art. Socialization: The student will engage in sharing and group cooperation during 75% of the opportunities given in art therapy groups. Positive Peer Interaction: The student will demonstrate appropriate interaction with peers during 80% of the opportunities given. Group Identity: The student will develop insight and an accurate perception of his/her behavior through group feedback and art experiences as measured by his/her behavior and content in artistic productions.

Note. Adapted from *Resource Packet for Art Therapists in Schools*, by the American Art Therapy Association (AATA). Copyright 1985 by the American Art Therapy Association (AATA). All rights reserved. Reprinted with permission from the American Art Therapy Association, Inc. (AATA).

diagnostic art therapy assessment were developed based upon the guidelines outlined by the American Art Therapy Association (1985). Table 5 highlights indicators for potential art therapy candidates. The list is used to assess the suitability of a student for a diagnostic art therapy assessment. If a student is found suitable, a recommendation for assessment is submitted with a rationale for a student's eligibility for art therapy services.

Silver Drawing Test (SDT)

The primary art therapy diagnostic assessment instrument administered to potential art therapy candidates in the Alternative Education Department at Monroe #1 BOCES was the Silver Drawing Test of Cognition and Emotion (1996) developed by Dr. Rawley Silver. The Silver Drawing Test (SDT) is written according to the Standards for Educational and Psychological Testing (AERA, APA, NCME, 1985). Silver (1996) states that the aim of the test is, "To provide an instrument for assessing the cognitive skills of individuals who have difficulty understanding others and making themselves understood" (p. 4). Silver (1996) identifies the four goals of the test:

1. To bypass language in evaluating the ability to solve conceptual problems.
2. To provide greater precision in evaluating cognitive strengths and weaknesses that might escape detection on verbal measures.
3. To facilitate the early identification of children or adolescents who may be depressed.
4. To provide a pre-post instrument for assessing progress or the effectiveness of educational or therapeutic programs.

The Silver Drawing Test (SDT) uses stimulus drawings to prompt response drawings that solve problems and represent concepts. Responses are scored on rating scales that range from 0 to 5 points, with 5 as the highest score. Silver (1996) points out scoring is based in part on experiments by Piaget and Inhelder (1967) and by Bruner and Associates (1966) who have traced the development of cognition through successive stages by presenting children with various tasks. The SDT includes three subtests: (1) Predictive Drawing, (2) Drawing from Observation, and (3) Drawing from Imagination. The SDT has two components: (1) cognitive, and (2) emotional.

The cognitive component deals with the three concepts identified by Piaget as fundamental in reading and mathematics: space, sequential order, and class inclusion. The SDT uses a visual-spatial approach

Table 5.
Indicators for Potential Art Therapy Candidates

Serious Emotional or Traumatic Experience Associated with Non-School Environment	Behavior Problems Manifested in School	Other Observable Manifestations of Behavior
• Crisis in Home • Death of Significant Other • Parental Separation, Divorce, or Remarriage • Serious Physical or Mental Illness • Physical or Psychological Abuse or Neglect • Substance Abuse	• Excessive Absences • Adjustment Difficulties • Peer Pressure • Poor Peer Interaction • Difficulty with Authority Figures • Academic Failure	• Chronically Irritable / Depressed / Angry • Withdrawn / Non-Verbal • Excessively Verbal / Over-Intellectual • Disruptive / Destructive / Aggressive • Poor Motivation • Insecure • Inappropriate Affect • Poor Body Image • Excessive Use of Fantasy • Expresses Self Through Art

Note. Adapted from *Resource Packet for Art Therapists in Schools*, by the American Art Therapy Association (AATA). Copyright 1985 by the American Art Therapy Association (AATA). All rights reserved. Reprinted with permission from the American Art Therapy Association, Inc. (AATA).

to testing these three concepts. The cognitive component is based on the theory that the SDT measures the ability to: (1) select, combine, and represent, (2) conserve and form a sequence, and (3) represent concepts of horizontality, verticality, height, width, and depth.

The emotional component is based on the theory that responses to the Drawing from Imagination task can provide access to fantasies and facilitate the early identification of children or adolescents who may be depressed or emotionally disturbed. Silver (1996) theorizes that a child who responds to the Drawing from Imagination task with a strongly negative theme or fantasy may be at risk for depression. Silver (1996) references the work of Aaron Beck and his associates (1979) on the cognitive view of clinical depression.

In discussing the cognitive view of unipolar depression, Ronald Comer (1995) asserts:

> Aaron Beck's research and clinical observations led him to believe that negative thinking . . . lies at the heart of unipolar depression. . . . He argues that depressed people are so filled with negative thoughts about themselves, their situations, and the future that all aspects of their functioning are affected dramatically. According to Beck, maladaptive attitudes, the cognitive triad, errors in thinking, and automatic thoughts combine to produce this pervasive negativity. (p. 286)

Maladaptive Attitudes

Beck (as cited in Comer, 1995) argues that children's attitudes toward themselves and the world are based on their own experiences, their family relationships, and the judgments of the people around them. The negative attitudes become templates, or schemas, against which the child evaluates every experience.

The Cognitive Triad

Beck (as cited in Comer, 1995) argues that negative thinking takes three forms, referred to as the cognitive triad. Individuals repeatedly interpret their experiences, themselves, and their futures in negative ways that lead them to feel depressed.

Errors in Thinking

Beck (as cited in Comer, 1995) argues that depressed people employ errors of logic or forms of distorted thinking, which helps to build and maintain the cognitive triad. These errors in logic include:

1. Arbitrary Inference: Drawing negative conclusions on the basis of little or even contrary evidence.
2. Selective Abstraction: Focusing on one negative detail of a situation while ignoring the larger context.
3. Overgeneralization: Drawing a broad conclusion from a single, perhaps insignificant event.
4. Minimization and Magnification: Underestimating the significance of positive experiences and exaggerating the significance of negative experiences.
5. Personalization: Incorrectly viewing the self as the cause of negative

events.

Automatic Thoughts

Beck (as cited in Comer, 1995) argues that depressed people experience the cognitive triad in the form of automatic thoughts, defined as a steady train of unpleasant thoughts that repeatedly remind them of their assumed inadequacy and the hopelessness of their situation.

The Silver Drawing Test (SDT) scale for assessing the emotional content of responses, called the Projection Scale, is based on the observation that respondents: (1) perceive the same stimulus drawings differently, (2) select stimulus drawings based on individual past experiences, and (3) selections trigger associations and fantasies expressed through drawings and stories. Silver (1996) states:

> It is theorized that responses to the Drawing from Imagination task reflect attitudes of the respondents toward themselves and toward others in ways that can be quantified. The score of 1 point is used to characterize strongly negative themes or fantasies; 2 points, to characterize moderately negative themes. . . . At the high end of the scale, 5 points is used to characterize strongly positive themes; 4 points, moderately positive. The neutral score, 3 points, is used for responses that are ambivalent, ambiguous, or unemotional. . . . Although this scale is a continuum ranging from strongly negative to strongly positive emotional content, it is not a progression from mental illness to mental health and should not be included in total SDT scores. When the scale is used as a pre-test and post-test, however, it can provide evidence of changes, such as regression or post-intervention progress. (pp. 17–18)

The age range recommended for the Silver Drawing Test (SDT) is from age 5 years to adult. There is no time limit for individual administration. In the scoring of the SDT, Silver (1996) cautions the scorer about combining subtest scores into total scores and the self-report requested in response to the Drawing from Imagination task. Silver (1996) explains:

> Some examinees receive low scores in some cognitive abilities, high scores in others. Consequently, their total score can mask particular strengths and weaknesses. . . . It has been found that self-reports are often unreliable and suggest resistance to disclosure. Nevertheless, they provide insight into masked depression, denial, and unconscious feelings, and can be useful when talking with respondents about their drawing. (p. 24)

The following additional diagnostic assessment instruments may also be administered to potential art therapy candidates:

House-Tree-Person Test (HTP)

John N. Buck developed the HTP in 1987. The purpose of the test is to provide information on personality characteristics and interpersonal relationships. There is no age limit and no time limit for individual administration. The examinee is asked to draw a House, a Tree, and a Person. The projective aspects of the HTP drawings include: (1) size, age, placement or presentation of the House, (2) kind, age, size, placement or presentation of the Tree, and (3) sex, facial expression, body stance, age, race, size, clothing, presentation or action of the Person. Scoring is based on the presence or absence of the various expressive aspects.

Kinetic House-Tree-Person Test (KHTP)

Robert C. Burns developed the KHTP in 1987. The purpose of the test is to introduce a kinetic or action component to the HTP, thereby increasing the amount of information available, both qualitatively and quantitatively within the drawing. There is no age limit and no time limit for administration. Examinees are presented a sheet of 8 ¹/₂ x 11 inch white paper placed horizontally and asked to "Draw a house, a tree, and a whole person on this paper with some kind of action." The projective aspects of the KHTP include attachment, distance, order, and size of figures in the drawings. In addition, different actions, styles, and symbols in the drawings are analyzed. Scoring is based on attachments that are present, figures other than self that are present, and additional figures that are present. Also noteworthy is the significance of which figure was drawn first.

Kinetic Family Drawings (KFD)

Robert C. Burns and S. Harvard Kaufman developed the KFD in 1972. The purpose of the KFD is to obtain information on self-concept and interpersonal relationships through the examinee's perception of the self in his or her family setting. Information is not only obtained about family dynamics but also the examinee's adaptive and defensive functioning. Examinees are presented with an 8 ¹/₂ x 11 inch sheet of plain white paper and a pencil and asked to "Draw a picture of everyone in your family, including you, DOING something." Interpretation of the KFD is based on the following: style, symbols, actions of individual figures, actions between individual figures, and characteristics of individual KFD figures. The use of the KFD grid sheet is also helpful in obtaining the measurements of the self and other KFD figures and the location of the self and the other figures.

Cognitive Art Therapy Assessment (CATA)

Dr. Ellen G. Horovitz developed the CATA in 1988. The purpose of the assessment is to compliment a multidisciplinary team's clinical findings with respect to developmental stages and personality facets of examinees. The assessment offers open-ended creative activities with pencil, paint, and clay. An essential source of information on specific kinds of behavior can be elicited through the utilization of the three different media. Line drawings elicit intellectually controlled expression and reality-based or fantasy-based storytelling. Paint elicits the expression of mood and affect. Clay elicits sustained efforts at constructive integration. There is no age limit and no time limit for individual administration. The directive to the examinee is "You have a choice to draw, paint, and make whatever you want from clay. You can do all three. With which (medium) would you like to start?" The interpretative aspects of the CATA include: (1) quality of the art work, (2) formal qualities of the art work, (3) subject matter, (4) attitude of the examinee, and (5) overall observations.

ART THERAPY APPLICATION

Theoretical Framework: Cognitive Model

The Cognitive Model is a theoretical perspective that emphasizes the process and content of thinking that underlies behavior. Cognitive therapy is based on a theory of personality, which maintains that how one thinks, largely determines how one feels and behaves. An individual's emotional and behavioral responses to a situation are largely determined by how that individual perceives, interprets, and assigns meaning to that situation. Raymond Corsini and Danny Wedding (1995) explain this theory of personality.

> Cognitive therapy views personality as shaped by the interaction between innate disposition and environment. Personality attributes are seen as reflecting basic schemas or interpersonal "strategies" developed in

response to the environment. Cognitive therapy sees psychological distress as being "caused" by a number of factors. While people may have biochemical predispositions to illness, they respond to specific stressors because of their learning history. . . . Individuals experience psychological distress when they perceive a situation as threatening their vital interests. At such times, their perceptions and interpretations of events are highly selective, egocentric, and rigid. This results in a functional impairment of normal cognitive activity ability. There is a decreased ability to turn off idiosyncratic thinking, to concentrate, recall, or reason. Corrective functions, which allow reality testing and refinement of global conceptualizations, are attenuated. (p. 236)

A variety of techniques may be used consistent with the cognitive model. Verbal techniques are used to elicit the patients/clients' thoughts, analyze the logic behind the thoughts, identify maladaptive assumptions, and examine the validity of those assumptions. Art therapy techniques are used to elicit the patients/clients' imagery as a pictorial representation of his or her cognitive distortions. The imagery is subjected to the same type of evaluation and modification as thoughts. Comer (1995) summarizes:

> To cognitive theorists, we are all artists who are both reproducing and creating our worlds in our mind as we try to understand the events going on around us. If we are effective artists, our cognitive representations tend to be accurate (agreed upon by others) and useful (adaptive). If we are ineffective artists, however, we may create a cognitive inner world that is alien to others and painful and harmful to ourselves. (p. 52)

Psychosocial Treatment

Treatment is the application of measures designed to alleviate a pathological condition. Psychosocial Treatment is the informed and systematic application of techniques based on established psychological principles, by professionals who are trained and experienced to understand these principles and to apply these techniques to modify feelings, thoughts, and behaviors deemed maladaptive.

With respect to psychosocial treatment in art therapy, Arthur Robbins and Linda Beth Sibley (1976) define an art therapy technique as, "A concrete implementation of theory introduced by the art therapist, at the appropriate time, to facilitate creative and therapeutic change" (p. 210). Robbins and Sibley (1976) explain that art therapy techniques can serve three separate purposes: (1) projective techniques are used for diagnosis; (2) research techniques are used to gather objective information; (3) therapeutic techniques are used to enhance communication in the therapeutic session. Robbins and Sibley (1976) caution, "Technique, however, is only one element of a network of component parts comprising the therapeutic situation. Technique can be no substitute for sensitivity to the specific patient/client population, relevant issues, goals, atmosphere, and setting" (p. 212).

The development challenges of adolescence coupled with the at-risk factors and the attitudes and personality characteristics of alternative education students underscore the need for effective therapeutic interventions. The following art therapy techniques provide the application of therapeutic art experiences with students at risk. The techniques, written in a lesson plan format, are designed to bridge not only the verbal and nonverbal, but also the logical and emotional. The photographic illustrations highlight the students' creative responses elicited from the therapeutic techniques. However, the focus is always on the process and not the product. It is the art therapy process, which allows the students at risk to explore their personal problems and potentials and find ways of making responsible choices.

As a precaution, the practitioner needs to be aware that the probable and possible topics raised as a result of introducing the techniques have the inherent potential for triggering a "hot cognition," or a powerful and highly meaningful thought or association that can produce strong emotional reactions. In the hands of skilled practitioners, the application of these techniques, in a safe and supportive environment, can help students review their problems and the options they have for dealing with them. Therefore, it is the responsibility of practitioners to take the appropriate professional precautions to ensure the safety and the psychological and emotional well being of students who participate in individual or group art therapy sessions. In addition, practitioners must be prepared to assist students in obtaining other therapeutic or supportive services if the problem or treatment is beyond the scope of practice of the practitioner.

ART THERAPY TECHNIQUES

- POETRY AS STIMULUS: POETRY'S IMAGES
  Focus: Insight

- MAGAZINE PHOTO COLLAGE: "GIFT" COLLAGES
  Focus: Acceptance

- LIFELINES
  Focus: Self-awareness

- INITIALS
  Focus: Self-awareness

- THEME CENTERED GROUP MURALS
  Focus: Group Dynamics

- JOURNALS
  Focus: Self-awareness

- THEME CENTERED GROUP MANDALAS
  Focus: Group Identity

- VOLCANO DRAWINGS
  Focus: Ventilation of Anger

- PERSONA AND ANIMA SELF-PORTRAITS
  Focus: Self-awareness

- BRIDGE DRAWINGS
  Focus: Self-awareness

- SYMBOLIC BANNERS
  Focus: Self-awareness

- MEDIA EXPLORATIONS
  Focus: Paint

- MANDALAS
  Focus: Self-awareness

- SELF-ASSESSMENTS : "THE GARDEN OF SELF"
  Focus: Self-awareness

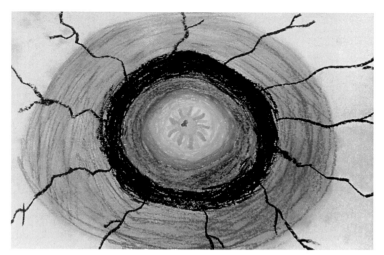

Figure 1. Poetry's Images.

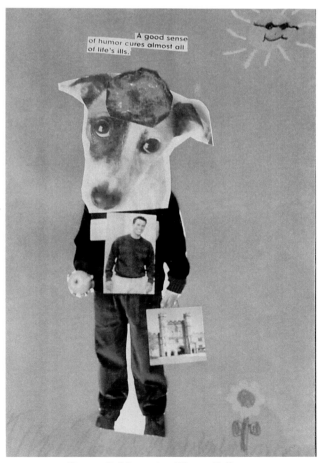

Figure 2. Magazine Photo Collage.

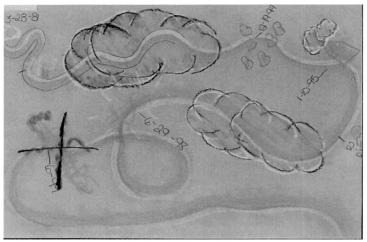

Figure 3. Lifelines.

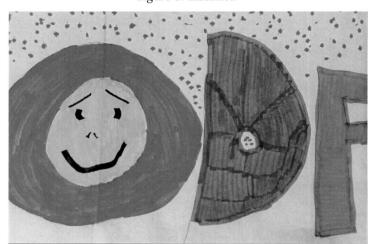

Figure 4. Initials.

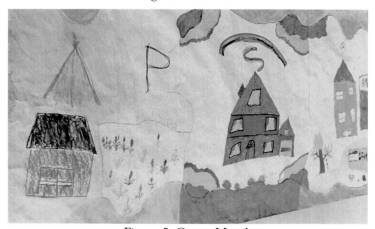

Figure 5. Group Mural

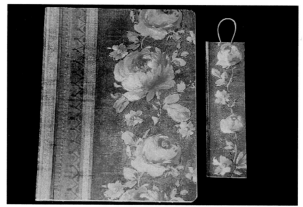

Figure 6. Journal.

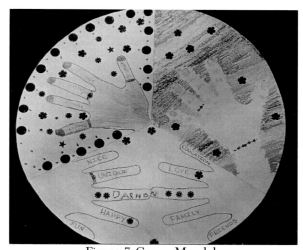

Figure 7. Group Mandala.

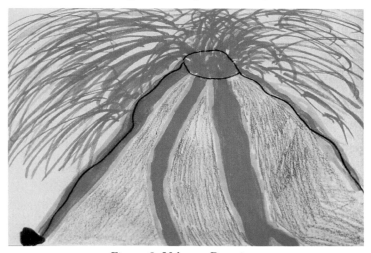

Figure 8. Volcano Drawing.

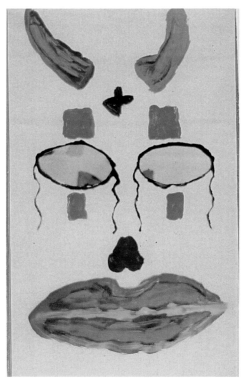

Figure 9. Persona and Anima Self-Portrait.

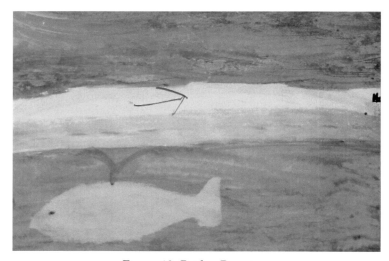

Figure 10. Bridge Drawing.

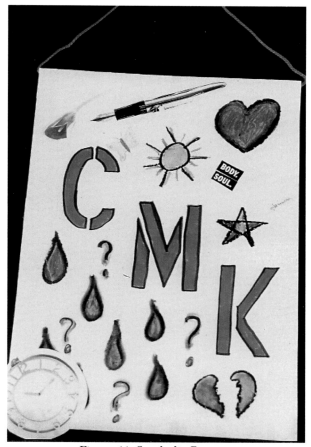

Figure 11. Symbolic Banner.

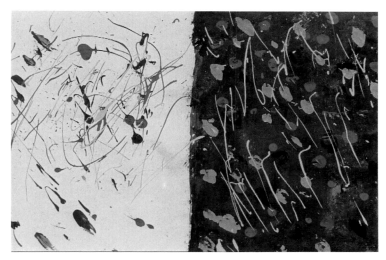

Figure 12. Media Exploration.

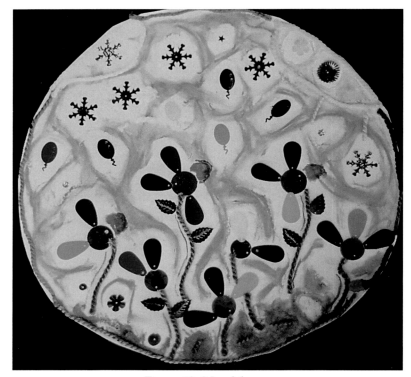

Figure 13. Mandala.

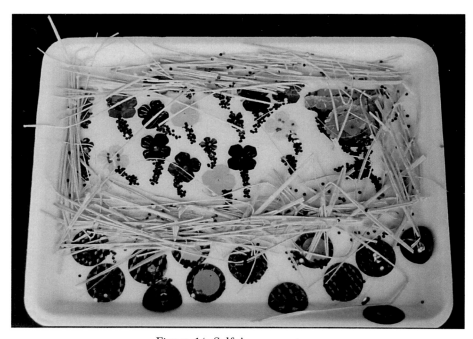

Figure 14. Self-Assessment.

TECHNIQUE: POETRY AS STIMULUS: POETRY'S IMAGES
(Figure 1)

FOCUS: Insight

OBJECTIVES:

1. To provide a structured opportunity for self-expression and communication.
2. To promote introspection and insight into thoughts and feelings.
3. To provide an opportunity to clarify feelings about the changing aspects of life.
4. To promote risk-taking through self-disclosure.
5. To promote empathy among group members.
6. To promote group identity and cohesion by providing an atmosphere for positive peer interaction.

MATERIALS:
1. Drawing Paper
   a. White
   b. Size: 12" x 18"
2. Assorted Drawing Media
   a. Colored Pencils
   b. Crayons
   c. Pastels
   d. Felt-tip Markers

DIRECTIONS:
1. Discuss Definitions:
   a. Poem:
      An arrangement of words written or spoken. Traditionally, a rhythmic composition, sometimes rhymed, expressing experiences, ideas, or emotions in a style more concentrated, imaginative, and powerful than that of ordinary speech or prose; some poems are in meter, some in free verse.
   b. Metaphor:
      A figure of speech in which the qualities of one thing are carried over to another thing. The metaphor always contains two parts, X and Y. The poet wants to create an equal sign between the two parts: X=Y.
2. Read the poem: The Story of Your Life
3. Ask the group members to individually create a

visual response to the poem.

4. Encourage each group member to share his or her creative response visually and verbally.

POPULATION: Adolescent Group
(12–18 years)

ISSUES: Probable and possible topics raised as a result of introducing this technique:

1. Ideas
2. Feelings
3. Perceptions about Self
4. Perceptions about Significant Others
5. Past Memories
6. Hurts or Joys of the Present
7. Fantasies of the Future
8. Alternative Choices of Behavior

THERAPIST: Harriet Wadeson
Modifications by Stella Stepney

THE STORY OF YOUR LIFE
by
Bruce Bennett

always a new wrinkle
a new corner a new alley
a new twist
to be revealed
to be explored
to be gone into
a new secret
a new outrage
to be exhumed to be excused
to be explained to be exonerated
oh always and always
it is endless and it is endlessly
fascinating
who would have thought who would have dreamed
who would have imagined
oh it is endless
and you go on and you go on and you go on
    and you go on
and never tire of it

Note. Reprinted with permission of Bruce Bennett.

TECHNIQUE: MAGAZINE PHOTO COLLAGE:
"GIFT" COLLAGES (Figure 2)

FOCUS: Acceptance

OBJECTIVES:

1. To promote an atmosphere for socialization and positive peer interaction.
2. To promote trust through risk-taking and sharing.
3. To develop insight about self-image by comparing self-image to other people's impressions and perceptions.
4. To understand the significance of personal traits and explore what qualities attract one person to another.
5. To allow group members to give and receive feedback.
6. To increase understanding and acceptance of others.

MATERIALS:

1. Drawing Paper
   a. White or Assorted Colors
   b. Size: 12" x 18"
2. Glue
3. Scissors
4. Pre-cut Magazine Images
5. Pencils or Markers to write comments

DIRECTIONS:

1. Distribute material to group members.
2. Ask each group member to think about the various qualities (traits or characteristics) that he or she likes in each of the individuals in the group (i.e., generous, creative, athletic) as well as other things that remind him or her about that person (i.e., colors, animals, music).
3. Ask the group members to look for pictures and words which represent each individual. (10 each)
4. After selecting the pictures and words, the group members give the images to each other.
5. When the group members have received the images from each person in the group, they may glue the pictures on the paper in any design to form a collage.

6. Encourage each group member to share his or her creative response by asking the following questions:
   a. How do you feel about the "gifts" you received?
   b. How did you feel about giving "gifts" to others?
   c. Is the collage an accurate representation of you?

POPULATION: Adolescent Group
(12–18 years)

ISSUES: Probable and possible topics raised as a result of introducing this technique:
1. Ideas
2. Feelings
3. Perceptions about Self
4. Perceptions about Others

THERAPIST: P. J. Furrer
Modifications by Stella Stepney

TECHNIQUE: LIFELINES (Figure 3)
FOCUS: Self-awareness
OBJECTIVES:

1. To provide an opportunity for self-disclosure and understand the significance of events and other people in the lives of group members.
2. To provide an opportunity to clarify feelings about the changing aspects of life.
3. To promote risk-taking through revealing negative aspects of one's own life.
4. To demonstrate universality through comparing life experiences and recognition of common problems.
5. To provide an opportunity to clarify feelings about what is missing from group members' lives and to identify stressful situations.
6. To recognize the potential to gain control over more aspects of group members' lives through the identification of personal strengths and weaknesses.

MATERIALS:
1. Drawing Paper
   a. White / Assorted Colors
   b. Size: 12" x 18"
2. Assorted Drawing Media
   a. Colored Pencils
   b. Crayons
   c. Pastels
   d. Felt-tip Markers

DIRECTIONS:
1. Discuss Definitions:
   a. Journey:
      Travel from one place to another.
   b. Road map:
      A course or path that is planned out in detail.
2. Ask each group member to draw his or her life as a line, journey, or road map, placing images and events along the way. The images may be drawn and/or written.
3. Encourage each group member to share his or her creative response visually and verbally.

POPULATION: Adolescent Group
(12–18 years)

ISSUES: Probable and possible topics raised as a result of introducing this technique:

1. Feelings
2. Perceptions about Self
3. Perceptions about Significant Others
4. Past Memories
5. Hurts or Joys of the Present
6. Space Attribution to Significant Events
7. Omissions
8. Cause and Effect Clarification
9. Patterns

THERAPIST: Janie Rhyne
Modifications by Stella Stepney

TECHNIQUE: INITIALS (Figure 4)
FOCUS: Self-awareness
OBJECTIVES:

1. To encourage creative and imaginative self-expression.
2. To provide an opportunity for group members to focus on individual visual awareness, to isolate parts from whole, and to recreate new wholes from the parts.
3. To produce a concrete representation of the creative process which can help build self-concept and positive feelings about abilities.
4. To involve group members in an enjoyable experience, which stimulates play and fantasy.
5. To enhance socialization and positive peer interaction.
6. To incorporate group feedback into self-evaluation.

MATERIALS:
1. Drawing Paper
   a. White
   b. Size: 12" x 18"
2. Assorted Drawing Media
   a. Colored Pencils
   b. Crayons
   c. Pastels
   d. Felt-tip Markers

DIRECTIONS:
1. Ask each group member to draw his or her own initials as large as possible on the drawing paper.
2. Ask the group to find suggested ideas for pictures, using their own initials and the design the initials make. Pictures may be realistic or abstract.
3. Explain that when they have discovered the picture, they may stay within the lines or go out of the lines, using as many colors as they wish.
4. Encourage each group member to share his or her creative response visually and verbally.

POPULATION: Adolescent Group
(12–18 years)

ISSUES: Probable and possible topics raised as a result of
                     introducing this technique:
                     1. Ideas
                     2. Individuality
                     3. Differences and Similarities
                     4. Feelings
                     5. Perceptions about Self
                     6. Perceptions about Others
THERAPIST: Helen Landgarten
                     Modifications by Stella Stepney

TECHNIQUE: THEME CENTERED GROUP MURALS
Fantasy Theme: "Life on an Island" (Figure 5)

FOCUS: Peer Group Dynamics

OBJECTIVES:

1. To use teamwork in the development of shared decision-making and task-performance.
2. To understand group dynamics and evaluate one's role in the group.
3. To share fantasies in order to promote a heightened awareness of self and others and explore the needs of others through the expression of wishes and desires.
4. To share viewpoints through the free exchange of ideas.
5. To allow members to give and receive feedback in a nonthreatening way.
6. To promote group identity and cohesion by bonding together and being supportive of one another.

MATERIALS:

1. Drawing Paper
   a. White
   b. Mural Size
2. Assorted Drawing Media
   a. Colored Pencils
   b. Crayons
   c. Pastels
   d. Felt-tip Markers

DIRECTIONS:

1. Ask the group to create a mural based on the fantasy theme, "Life on an Island."
2. Explain that each group member should have a designated space on the paper to draw anything he or she wishes to draw.
3. Upon completion of the mural ask the group:
   a. How they felt about the mural?
   b. How they felt during the process of creating the mural?
   c. How they felt about the art experience?

POPULATION: Adolescent Group
(12–18 Years)

ISSUES: Group Dynamics:

1. How does the art form get started?
2. Who takes the initiative?
3. Whose suggestions were used? Ignored?
4. Do people take turns, form teams or work simultaneously?
5. Is anyone left out?
6. Where are the locations of each person's work and how much space is used by each person?
7. Do people add to others' work?
8. Who is the leader or most active participant?
9. Who is the scapegoat?
10. Was it an enjoyable or threatening experience?

THERAPIST: Marian Liebmann
               Modifications by Stella Stepney

TECHNIQUE: JOURNALS: Recording Experiences and Reflections (Figure 6)

FOCUS: Self-awareness

OBJECTIVES:

1. To promote introspection, insight, and the expression of moods, feelings, and ideas.
2. To promote reminiscence.
3. To identify feelings of discomfort and ventilate fears and anxiety.
4. To identify issues, feelings of concern, and stressful situations.
5. To recognize the causes and appropriateness of moods and emotions.
6. To explore imagination in order to arrive at generalized perceptions about oneself.

MATERIALS:

1. Composition Books
2. Wallpaper Samples
3. Scissors
4. Glue

DIRECTIONS:

1. Discuss Emotion:
   Feeling state with mind, body, and behavioral components.
2. Brainstorm a list of emotions with group members.
3. Ask group members to identify a recently experienced emotion. Ask the group to consider these questions:
   a. Was the feeling pleasant?
   b. Was the feeling unpleasant?
   c. What caused the feeling?
   d. Are there any patterns?
   e. How are you feeling now?
3. Discuss Journals:
   A journal is a personal record of one's experiences and reflections. Journals enable individuals to become aware of their feelings.
   a. Feelings can be expressed as symbols.
   b. Feelings can be expressed in stories or poetry.
   c. Feelings can be expressed through doodles or sketches.

d. Feelings can be expressed in letter writing.

e. Feelings can be expressed by making lists: things to do, goals, accomplishments, friends, enemies, strength, weaknesses, or favorites, etc.

4. Ask each group member to select a wallpaper sample to cover the front, back, and inside of the composition book.

5. Encourage each group member to use the journal as a tool to increase self-awareness.

POPULATION: Adolescent Group
               (12–18 years)
ISSUES: Probable and possible topics raised as a result of introducing this technique:
               1. Feelings
               2. Perceptions about Self
               3. Perceptions about Significant Others
               4. Past Memories
               5. Hurts or Joys of the Present
               6. Patterns
               7. Fantasies of the Future
THERAPIST: Harriet Wadeson
               Modifications by Stella Stepney

TECHNIQUE: THEME CENTERED GROUP MANDALAS
                      Theme: "Mandala of Hands" (Figure 7)

FOCUS: Peer Group Identity

OBJECTIVES:

1. To build trust and promote group identity and cohesion in order to create a supportive group environment.
2. To provide an opportunity for each group member to focus on his or her visual awareness, to isolate parts from wholes, and to recreate new wholes from the parts.
3. To produce a concrete representation of the creative process, which can build self-concept and positive feelings about abilities.
4. To compare different interpretations and perspectives in order for group members to learn more about each other.
5. To encourage social interaction and gain insight about interpersonal behavior.
6. To promote recognition of the common bond among group members.

MATERIALS:

1. Compass or Template to be used for tracing circles.
2. Drawing Paper
   a. White
   b. Size: 18" x 24"
3. Assorted Drawing Media
   a. Colored Pencils
   b. Crayons
   c. Pastels
   d. Felt-tip Markers
4. Assorted Collage Material
   a. Glitter
   b. Sequins
   c. Buttons

DIRECTIONS:

1. Draw a circle approximately 18" in diameter.
2. Divide the circle into segments based upon the number of group members.
3. Define Mandala:
   A mandala, which is the Sanskrit word for

"circle," is a universal art form. The mandala is a balanced, centered design executed within a circular context.

4. Distribute one segment of the circle to each group member.
5. Ask group members to trace the outline of his or her hand anywhere inside the segment.
6. Ask group members to imaginatively and creatively design his or her segment.
7. Encourage each group member to share his or her creative response visually and verbally.
8. Ask group members to combine their segments to create a group mandala.

POPULATION: Adolescent Group
                  (12–18 Years)

ISSUES: Probable and possible topics raised as a result of introducing this technique:
1. Perception of Self
2. Perception of Group
3. Group Identity and Cohesion
4. Trust
5. Support
6. Risk-taking

THERAPIST: Marian Liebmann
                  Modifications by Stella Stepney

TECHNIQUE: VOLCANO DRAWINGS (Figure 8)
FOCUS: Ventilation: Projecting Anger
OBJECTIVES:

1. To provide an opportunity to express feelings of anger and frustration.
2. To promote an awareness of environmental influences and stimulation in order to recognize feelings as a response to the environment.
3. To provide the opportunity for mutual self-disclosure and encourage empathy through identification with feelings of others.
4. To promote interpersonal learning through sharing constructive responses to negative experiences.
5. To identify appropriate methods of dealing with anger.
6. To develop new coping strategies.

MATERIAL:

1. Drawing Paper
   a. White
   b. Size 12" x 18"
2. Assorted Drawing Media
   a. Colored Pencils
   b. Crayons
   c. Pastels
   d. Felt-tip Markers

DIRECTIONS:

1. Define Anger:
   A negative internal feeling state associated with specific cognitive and perceptual distortions and deficiencies, subjective labeling, physiological changes, and action tendencies to engage in socially constructed and reinforced organized behavior scripts.
2. Introduce the idea that at times, situations can make individuals feel angry and that people express their anger experiences differently.
3. Discuss the various ways people choose to deal with, avoid, or channel their anger.
4. Discuss the concept of a volcano as a metaphor for anger. A volcano is an opening in the earth's crust through which molten lava, ash, and gases

are ejected. The volcano can be viewed as a symbol that represents a dichotomy of tension and distension: (1) whether to release, (2) when to release, and (3) how to release.

5. Ask each group member to think about a particular situation that has made him or her experience feelings of anger. Then, ask each member to create a "personal" volcano based upon the expressed feeling.

6. When drawings are completed, ask each member to:
   a. Give the drawing a title.
   b. Write a paragraph about the situation, including how he or she dealt with the situation.

7. Group Discussion:
   a. Have each member share his or her creative response visually and verbally.
   b. Encourage group members to suggest ways that each presenter could have dealt constructively with the situation.

POPULATION: Adolescent Group
(12 –18 years)

ISSUES: Probable and possible topics raised as a result of introducing this technique:
1. Anger Triggers
2. Perceptions about Self
3. Perceptions about Others
4. Past Memories
5. Alternative Choices of Behavior

THERAPIST: Carol Cox
Modifications by Stella Stepney

TECHNIQUE: PERSONA and ANIMA SELF-PORTRAITS
(Figure 9)

FOCUS: Self-awareness

OBJECTIVES:

1. To encourage projection of self-image and explore feelings of self-evaluation.
2. To promote risk-taking through revealing positive and negative aspects of one's own life.
3. To promote feedback about perceptions of self and others.
4. To incorporate group feedback into self-evaluation.
5. To develop insight about self-image.
6. To develop group cohesion through mutual self disclosure.

MATERIALS:

1. Assorted Media for Masks
   a. Full-Face or Half-Face Pre-formed White Masks
      (1) Plaster
      (2) Plastic
      (3) Foam
   b. Paper Bags: 6" x 10" or 12" x 17"
      (1) Brown
      (2) White
2. Assorted Drawing Media
   a. Colored Pencils
   b. Crayons
   c. Pastels
   d. Felt-tip Markers
3. Assorted Paint Media
   a. Acrylic
   b. Tempera
4. Assorted Collage Material
   a. Sequins
   b. Glitter

DIRECTIONS:

1. Define the term Persona:
   A mask or way of appearing that is appropriate to a specific role or social setting. It both shields an individual and reveals suitable aspects of the personality, but is often at variance with the personality as a whole. In essence, it is the outside or social self that a person presents to the world.

2. Define the term Anima:
   That part of the personality, which is in close contact with the unconscious. It serves as a bridge to the unconscious in both men and women. In essence, it is the inner or private self.
3. Ask the group members to depict their persona or outside self on the outside of the mask. The outside should represent the way he or she presents him or her self to others and how he or she personally feels others see him or her.
4. Ask the group members to depict their anima or inside self on the inside of the mask. The inside should represent the thoughts, feelings, and images that are not readily accessible to others.
5. Encourage each group member to share his or her creative response visually and verbally.

POPULATION: Adolescent Group
              (12–18 years)
ISSUES: Probable and possible topics raised as a result of introducing this technique:
             1. Perceptions about Self
             2. Perceptions about Significant Others
             3. Ideas
             4. Feelings
             5. Past Memories
             6. Hurts or Joys of the Present
             7. Fantasies of the Future
THERAPIST: Harriet Wadeson
             Modifications by Stella Stepney

TECHNIQUE:	BRIDGE DRAWINGS (Figure 10)
FOCUS:	Self-awareness
OBJECTIVES:	

1. To provide an opportunity for self-disclosure and for the exploration of individual significant concerns.
2. To compare different interpretations and perspectives in order to heighten awareness of self and others.
3. To promote introspection and insight and explore feelings of self-evaluation.
4. To recognize personal strengths and weaknesses.
5. To share feelings and fears about adjusting to change.
6. To explore ways of overcoming personal conflicts, problems, and obstacles.

MATERIALS:
1. Drawing Paper
   a. White
   b. Size: 12" x 18"
2. Assorted Drawing Media
   a. Colored Pencils
   b. Crayons
   c. Pastels
   d. Felt-tip Markers

DIRECTIONS:
1. Define Bridge:
   A structure spanning and providing passage over an obstacle.
2. Ask group members to draw a picture of a bridge going from someplace to someplace.
3. After completing the drawing, ask group members to indicate with an arrow the direction of travel.
   Left: ⟵
   Right: ⟶
4. Ask group members to place a dot (.) to indicate where they see themselves in the picture.
5. Encourage each group member to share his or her creative response visually and verbally.

POPULATION: Adolescent Group
(12–18 years)

ISSUES: Probable and possible topics raised as a result of introducing this technique.
1. Adolescence as a transition phase between childhood and adulthood.
2. Exploration of identity and independence as the developmental tasks of adolescence.
3. Interpretative variables specific to the Bridge Drawing:
   a. Directionality:
      The arrow is used to indicate the direction of travel when crossing the bridge. The left side is considered the past, the right side is considered the future, and the direction of travel would be from the past to the future.
      Past: ⟵
      Future: ⟶
   b. Placement of self in the picture:
      The placement of the dot (.) to represent the self indicates the distance ahead in crossing the bridge as well as the distance that has been traveled. This reveals how the adolescent sees himself or herself in relationship to a goal or solution to a problem.
   c. Places drawn on either side of the bridge:
      The places or landmasses drawn on either side of the bridge may indicate a specific goal to be reached.
      (1) Named Places or Landmasses
      (2) Unnamed Places or Landmasses
      (3) Symbolic Connections
   d. Emphasis by elaboration:
      The elaboration in the drawing will show where the most emphasis is placed—in the past, in the future, or on the bridge itself.
   e. Matter drawn under the bridge:
      The matter drawn under the bridge will either be perceived as threatening or nonthreatening in nature.

THERAPISTS: Ronald Hays and Sherry Lyons
              Modifications by Stella Stepney

TECHNIQUE: SYMBOLIC BANNERS (Figure 11)
FOCUS: Self-awareness
OBJECTIVES:

1. To provide an opportunity for self-disclosure.
2. To highlight personal qualities (traits or characteristics) and reveal oneself through the choice of symbols that represent those qualities.
3. To promote insight.
4. To explore imagination in order to arrive at a generalized perception of oneself.
5. To promote feedback about perceptions of self and others.
6. To increase understanding and acceptance of self and others.

MATERIALS:
1. Drawing Paper
   a. White
   b. Size 12" x 18"
2. Assorted Drawing Media
   a. Colored Pencils
   b. Crayons
   c. Pastels
   d. Felt-tip Markers
3. Assorted Paint Media
   a. Acrylic
   b. Tempera
   c. Watercolor
4. Pre-cut Magazine Images
5. Glue
6. Craft Sticks
7. Yarn
8. Glitter
9. Sequins
10. Buttons
11. Feathers

DIRECTIONS:
1. Define Symbol:
   Any object that represents another object.
2. Define Symbolism:
   Use of symbols.
3. Introduce the concept of symbols as vehicles of communication that allow individuals and/or

groups to represent what they want people to know about them.
   a. Flags
   b. Insignias
   c. Coats of Arms
   d. Badges
   e. Banners
4. Ask group members to think about what they would like other people to know about them.
   a. What would their personal symbols look like?
   b. What images or colors would they use?
5. Ask group members to design a personal symbolic banner.
6. Encourage each group member to share his or her creative response visually and verbally.

POPULATION: Adolescent Group
             (12–18 Years)
ISSUES: Probable and possible topics raised as a result of introducing this technique:
             1. Perceptions about Self
             2. Self-esteem
             3. Identity
             4. Ideas
             5. Feelings
             6. Memories of the Past
             7. Joys of the Present
             8. Fantasies of the Future
THERAPIST: Marian Liebmann
             Modifications by Stella Stepney

TECHNIQUE: MEDIA EXPLORATIONS (Figure 12)
FOCUS: Paint Media
OBJECTIVES:

    1. To explore a variety of paint media and the elements of color, form, shape, and texture.
    2. To use the medium of paint to explore the realm of feeling and emotion through color.
    3. To experience pleasure and increase knowledge of emotion.
    4. To build perception skills.
    5. To communicate through images and explore personal associations.
    6. To encourage and reinforce creative and imaginative self-expression, which can build self-concept and positive feelings about abilities.

MATERIALS:
    1. Assorted Paint Media
       a. Acrylic
       b. Tempera
       c. Watercolor
    2. Assorted Paper
       a. Construction
       b. Paper Canvas
       c. Watercolor
    3. Assortment of Brushes
    4. Palettes
    5. Water
    6. Containers
    7. Cleaning Cloths / Paper Towels
    8. Protective Clothing

DIRECTIONS:
    1. Introduce paint using primary and secondary colors.
    2. Allow group members to experiment with the variety of paint and paint textures to learn the behaviors of the paint.
    3. Ask group members to create an abstract or representational painting.
    4. Encourage group members to share his or her creative response visually and to verbally express his or her reactions to the painting experience to discern what feelings were evoked by

the colors that were used.

POPULATON: Adolescent Group
              (12–18 Years)

ISSUES: Probable and possible topics raised as a result of
              introducing this technique:
              1. Perceptions about Self
              2. Ideas
              3. Feelings
              4. Symbols
              5. Memories / Experiences
              6. Metaphors
              7. Fantasies

THERAPIST: Marian Liebmann
              Modifications by Stella Stepney

TECHNIQUE: MANDALAS (Figure 13)
FOCUS: Self-awareness
OBJECTIVES:

1. To create a balanced centered design for contemplation and reflection.
2. To promote self-disclosure.
3. To promote introspection and insight.
4. To build perception skills.
5. To communicate through images and explore personal associations.
6. To incorporate group feedback into self-evaluation.

MATERIALS:

1. Compass or Template to be used for tracing circles.
2. Drawing Paper
   a. White
   b. Size: 18" x 24"
3. Assorted Drawing Media
   a. Colored Pencils
   b. Crayons
   c. Pastels
   d. Felt-tip Markers
4. Assorted Paint Media
   a. Acrylic
   b. Tempera
   c. Watercolor
5. Assorted Collage Material
6. Paint brushes, palettes, water, and containers
7. Glue

DIRECTIONS:

1. Draw circles approximately 18" in diameter.
2. Define Mandala:
   A mandala, which is the Sanskrit word for "circle," is a universal art form. The mandala is a balanced, centered design executed within a circular context.
3. Distribute one circle to each group member.
4. Ask group members to create an abstract or representational design within the circle.
5. Encourage each group member to share his or her creative response visually and verbally.

POPULATION: Adolescent Group
(12–18 Years)

ISSUES: Probable and possible topics raised as a result of introducing this technique:
1. Perception of Self
2. Ideas
3. Feelings
4. Symbols
5. Metaphors
6. Fantasies

THERAPIST: Judith Cornell
Modifications by Stella Stepney

TECHNIQUE: SELF ASSESSMENTS: "The Garden of Self"
(Figure 14)

FOCUS: Self-awareness

OBJECTIVES:

1. To provide an opportunity for self-disclosure.
2. To promote introspection and insight.
3. To explore feelings of self-evaluation.
4. To recognize personal strengths and weaknesses.
5. To identify and interpret individual needs.
6. To identify personal goals.

MATERIALS:

1. Assorted Drawing Media
   a. Colored Pencils
   b. Crayons
   c. Pastels
   d. Felt-tip Markers
2. Assorted Paint Media
   a. Acrylic
   b. Tempera
3. Assorted Collage Material
   a. Cut Paper
   b. Found Objects
   c. Magazine Pictures / Words
   d. Tissue Paper
   e. Wallpaper Samples
4. Miscellaneous
   a. Drawing Paper
   b. Styrofoam Trays
   c. Glue
   d. Craft Sticks
   e. Glitter
   f. Pipe Cleaners
   g. Yarn

DIRECTIONS:

1. Define Garden:
   A plot of land used for growing flowers, vegetables, herbs, or fruit. A fertile, well-cultivated garden requires the right mixture of soil, water, and sunlight. Gardening offers many challenges, surprises, frustrations, and rewards.
2. Introduce the concept of a garden with three distinct categories: (1) healthy plants, (2) choking weeds, and (3) seeds.

3. Ask the group members to design a "Garden of Self" based on the concept of healthy plants, choking weeds, and seeds. As metaphors:

    a. The healthy plants represent the positive strengths and attributes the individual possesses.

    b. The choking weeds represent the issues or problems in living that can potentially inhibit growth and development.

       (1) Relational Problems

       (2) Problems Related to Abuse or Neglect

       (3) Academic Problems

       (4) Occupational Problems

       (5) Identity Problems

       (6) Acculturation Problems

       (7) Bereavement

    c. The seeds represent personal goals for the future.

4. Encourage each group member to share his or her creative response visually and verbally.

POPULATION: Adolescent Group
(12–18 years)

ISSUES: Probable and possible topics raised as a result of introducing this technique:
1. Personal Strengths or Positive Attributes
2. Issues or Problems in Living
3. Personal Goals

THERAPIST: Sandra Ticen
Modifications by Stella Stepney

REFERENCES

Allen, P. B. (1995). *Art is a Way of Knowing.* Boston, MA: Shambhala Publications, Inc.

Alschuler, R. H., & Hattwick, L. (1969). *Painting and Personality: A Study of Young Children.* Chicago, IL: The University of Chicago Press.

American Art Therapy Association. (1985). *Art Therapy in the Schools: A Position Paper of the American Art Therapy Association.* Mundelein, IL: Author.

American Art Therapy Association. (1985). *Resource Packet for Art Therapists in Schools.* Mundelein, IL: Author.

American Art Therapy Association. (1990). Art Therapy: Definition of the Profession. *Newsletter of the American Art Therapy Association,* Vol. 23, No. 1, 3.

American Art Therapy Association. (1997). Title and Scope of Practice. Mundelein, IL: Author.

American Art Therapy Association. (2001). *Ethics Document.* Mundelein, IL: Author.

American Educational Research Association, American Psychological Association, & National Council on Measurements in Education. (1985). *Standards for Educational and Psychological Testing.* Washington, DC: American Psychological Association.

Anderson, F. E. (1992). *Art for all the Children: Approaches to Art Therapy for Children with Disabilities.* (2nd ed.). Springfield, IL: Charles C Thomas.

Axline, V. M. (1969). *Play Therapy.* New York: Ballantine Books.

Beck, A. T. (1967). *Depression: Clinical, Experimental and Theoretical Aspects.* New York: Harper & Row.

Beck, A. T., Rush, J., Shaw, B. F., & Emory, G. (1979). *Cognitive Theory of Depression.* New York: Guilford Press.

Beck, A. T. (1991). Cognitive Therapy: A 30-year Retrospective. *American Psychology,* Vol. 46, No. 4, 368–375.

Bennett, B. (2001). *Personal Communication.*

Brendtro, L., Brokenleg, M., & Van Bockern, S. (1998). *Reclaiming Youth At Risk: Our Hope for the Future.* Bloomington, IN: National Educational Services.

Brooke, S. L. (1996). *A Therapist's Guide to Art Therapy Assessments.* Springfield, IL: Charles C Thomas.

Brooke, S. L. (1997). *Art Therapy with Sexual Abuse Survivors.* Springfield, IL: Charles C Thomas.

Buck, J. N. (1987). *The House-Tree-Person Technique: Revised Manual.* Los Angeles, CA: Western Psychological Services.

Bullis, R. (1984). *Spirituality in Social Work Practice.* Washington, DC: Taylor & Francis.

Burns, R. C. (1987). *Kinetic-House-Tree-Person Drawings: An Interpretative Manual.* New York: Brunner/Mazel, Inc.

Burns, R. C., & Kaufman, S. H. (1972). *Actions, Styles, and Symbols in Kinetic Family Drawings.* New York: Brunner/Mazel, Inc.

Bush, J. (1997). *The Handbook of School Art Therapy.* Springfield, IL: Charles C Thomas.

Campbell, D. (1997). *The Mozart Effect: Tapping the Power of Music to Heal the Body, Strengthen the Mind, and Unlock the Creative Spirit.* New York: Avon Books.

Cane, F. (1983). *The Artist in Each of Us.* Craftsbury Commons, VT: Art Therapy Publications.

Canfield, J., Hansen, M. V., & Kirberger, K. (1998). *Chicken Soup for the Teenage Soul Journal.* Deerfield Beach, FL: Health Communications, Inc.

Carrell, S. (1993). *Group Exercises for Adolescents: A Manual for Therapists.* Newbury Park, CA: SAGE Publications, Inc.

Chaplin, J. P. (1985). *Dictionary of Psychology* (2nd ed.). New York: Dell Publishing Co.

Cohen, B. M., Barnes, M. M., & Rankin, A. B. (1995). *Managing Traumatic Stress Through Art: Drawing from the Center.* Lutherville, MD: The Sidran Press.

Comer, R. J. (1995). *Abnormal Psychology* (2nd ed.). New York: W. H. Freeman & Co.

Corey, M. S., & Corey, G. (1997). *Groups: Process and Practice* (5th ed.). Pacific Grove, CA: Brooks/Cole Publishing Company.

Cornell, J. (1994). *Mandala: Luminous Symbols for Healing.* Wheaton, IL: The Theosophical Publishing House.

Corsini, R. J., & Wedding, D. (Eds.). 1995. *Current Psychotherapies* (5th ed.). Itasca, IL: F. E. Peacock Publisher, Inc.

Dunning, S., & Stafford, W. (1992). *Getting the Knack: 20 Poetry Writing Exercises.* Urbana, IL: National Council of Teachers of English.

Egan, G. (1998). *The Skilled Helper: A Problem-Management Approach to Helping.* Pacific Grove, CA: Brooks/Cole Publishing Company.

Frank, J. D., & Frank, J. B. (1991). *Persuasion & Healing: A Comparative Study of Psychotherapy* (3rd ed.). Baltimore, MD: The John Hopkins University Press.

Fryrear, J. L., & Corbit, I. E. (1992). *Photo Art Therapy: A Jungian Perspective.* Springfield, IL: Charles C Thomas.

Fuller, C. G., & Sabatino, D. A. (1996). Who Attends Alternative High Schools? *The High School Journal,* Vol. 79, No. 4, 293–297.

Furrer, P. J. (1982). *Art Therapy Activities and Lesson Plans for Individuals and Groups.* Springfield, IL: Charles C Thomas.

Hammer, E. F. (1958). *The Clinical Application of Projective Drawings* (6th Printing, 1980). Springfield, IL: Charles C Thomas.

Hays, R. E., & Lyons, S.J. (1981). The Bridge Drawing: A Projective Technique For Assessment in Art Therapy. *The Arts in Psychotherapy,* Vol. 8, 207–217, Ankho International Inc.

Horovitz-Darby, E. G. (1988). Art therapy assessment of a minimally language skilled deaf child. Proceedings from the 1988 University of California's Center on Deafness Conference: *Mental Health Assessment of Deaf Clients: Special Conditions.* Little Rock, AK: ADARA.

Horovitz-Darby, E. G. (1994). *Spiritual Art Therapy: An Alternate Path.* Springfield, IL: Charles C Thomas.

Horovitz, E. G. (1999). *A Leap of Faith: The Call to Art.* Springfield, IL: Charles C Thomas.

Kaplan, H. I., & Sadock, B. J. (1991). *Comprehensive Glossary of Psychiatry and Psychology.* Baltimore, MD: Williams & Wilkins.

Landgarten, H.B. (1981). *Clinical Art Therapy: A Comprehensive Guide.* New York: Brunner/Mazel, Publishers.

Landgarten, H. B. (1993). *Magazine Photo Collage: A Multicultural Assessment and Treatment Technique.* New York: Brunner/Mazel, Publishers.

Liebmann, M. (1986). *Art Therapy for Groups: A Handbook of Themes, Games, and Exercises.* Cambridge, MA: Brookline Books.

Linesch, D. (1988). *Adolescent Art Therapy.* New York: Brunner/Mazel, Publishers.

Linesch, D. (Ed.). (1993). *Art Therapy with Families in Crisis: Overcoming Resistance Through Nonverbal Expression.* New York: Brunner/Mazel, Publishers.

Lukas, S. (1993). *Where to Start and What to Ask: An Assessment Handbook.* New York: W. W. Norton & Company.

Malchiodi, C. A. (1997). *Breaking the Silence: Art Therapy with Children from Violent Homes.* Bristol, PA: Brunner/Mazel, Publishers.

Masterson, J. F. (1988). *The Search for the Real Self.* New York: The Free Press.

Maxmen, J. S., & Ward, N. G. (1995). *Essential Psychopathology and Its Treatment* (2nd edition Revised for DSM-IV). New York: W. W. Norton & Company.

McGoldrick, M., & Gerson, R. (1985). *Genograms in Family Assessment.* New York: W. W. Norton & Company.

McNiff, S. (1992). *Art as Medicine: Creating Therapy of the Imagination.* Boston: Shambhala.

McNiff, S. (1998). *Art-Based Research.* London, England: Jessica Kingsley Publisher Ltd.

Miller, A. (1997). *The Drama of the Gifted Child: The Search for the True Self.* New York: Basic Books.

Miller, J. B., & Stiver, I. P. (1997). *The Healing Connection: How Women Form Relationships in Therapy and in Life.* Boston, MA: Beacon Press.

Moon, B. L. (1995). *Existential Art Therapy: The Canvas Mirror* (2nd ed.). Springfield, IL: Charles C Thomas.

Morganett, R. S. (1990). *Skills for Living: Group Counseling Activities for Young Adolescents.* Champaign, IL: Research Press.

Morrison, M. R. (Ed.). (1987). *Poetry as Therapy.* New York: Human Sciences Press, Inc.

Naumburg, M. (1966). *Dynamically Oriented Art Therapy: Its Principles and Practice.* New York: Grune & Stratton, Inc.

Naumburg, M. (1973). *An Introduction to Art Therapy: Studies of the "Free" Art Expression of Behavior Problem Children and Adolescents as a Means of Diagnosis and Therapy.* New York: Teachers College Press.

Orleman, J. (1998). *Telling Secrets: An Artist's Journey Through Childhood Trauma.* Washington, DC: Child Welfare League of America, Inc.

Penaloza, J. (2000). Personal Communication.

Radgett, R. (Ed.). (1987). *The Teachers & Writers Handbook of Poetic Forms.* New York: Teachers & Writers Collaborative.

Rampersad, A., & Roessel, D. (Eds.). (1994). *The Collected Poems of Langston Hughes.* New York: Vintage Books.

Riley, S. (1999). *Contemporary Art Therapy with Adolescents.* London, England: Jessica Kingsley Publishers Ltd.

Robbins, A., & Sibley, L. B. (1976). *Creative Art Therapy.* New York: Brunner/Mazel, Publishers.

Robbins, A. (1994). *A Multi-Modal Approach to Creative Art Therapy.* London, England: Jessica Kingsley Publishers Ltd.

Ross, C. (1997). *Something to Draw On: Activities and Interventions Using an Art Therapy*

Approach. London, England: Jessica Kingsley Publishers Ltd.

Rubin, J. A. (Ed.). (1987). *Approaches to Art Therapy: Theory and Technique.* New York: Brunner/Mazel, Inc.

Shirk, S. R. (Ed.). (1988). *Cognitive Development and Child Psychotherapy.* New York: Plenum Press.

Silver, R. A. (1996). *Silver Drawing Test of Cognition and Emotion.* Sarasota, FL: Ablin Press Distributors.

Spring, D. (1993). *Shattered Images: Phenomenological Language of Sexual Trauma.* Chicago, IL: Magnolia Street Publishers.

Statt, D. (1986). *Dictionary of Psychology.* New York: Barnes & Noble Books.

Ticen, S. (2000). Personal Communication.

Wadeson, H. (1980). *Art Psychotherapy.* New York: John Wiley & Sons, Inc.

Wadeson, H. (Ed.). (1992). *A Guide to Conducting Art Therapy Research.* Mundelein, IL: American Art Therapy Association, Inc.

Williams, G. H., & Wood, M. M. (1995). *Developmental Art Therapy.* Baltimore, MD: University Park Press.

Yalom, I. D. (1975). *The Theory and Practice of Group Psychotherapy* (2nd ed.). New York: Basic Books.

Yalom, I. D. (1983). *Inpatient Group Psychotherapy.* New York: Basic Books.

Chapter 7

CONCLUSION

EDUCATIONAL THEORISTS have identified four ecological hazards in the lives of at-risk adolescents. The hazards include destructive relationships, climates of futility, learned irresponsibility, and loss of purpose.

Metaphorically, the concept of the "Garden of Self" composed of healthy plants, weeds, and seeds can be applied to art therapy with students who are at risk. The growth of these healthy adolescents is being stunted and choked out by academic, behavioral, and social weeds. Therefore, seeds of encouragement must be planted into the lives of these adolescents, which will enable them to not only master the developmental tasks of adolescence but also be successful in school.

During my experience in working with the Alternative Education Department, I was introduced to a philosophical and theoretical framework that calls for a reclaiming of youth at risk. To reclaim is to recover and redeem, to restore value to something that has been devalued. The reclaiming environment is one that creates changes that meet the needs of both the young person and the society. The theorists propose that belonging, mastery, independence, and generosity are the central values or the unifying theme of positive cultures for education and youth-work programs. The theorists conceive this philosophy as being embodied in a "Circle of Courage."

The concept of a "Circle of Courage" provides a unique perspective for working with at-risk populations. It is believed that successful individuals who work with children and adolescents at risk are those who can reframe cognition to foster the positive feelings and actions essential to the helping process. This is accomplished by employing esteeming labels, where positive traits are attributed to children and adolescents, coupled with empathizing labels, where cause is attributed to the situation.

With respect to the relationship between learning and mental health, art therapy with students who are at risk is a reframing of their cognition. Art therapy provides the positive cognitive, emotional, and social growth fostering opportunities for creative self-expression that can enhance the student's consciousness of self, others, and the environment. In essence, art therapy is a frame of mind.

"He who learns, teaches."
(Ancient African Proverb)

REFERENCE

Brendtro, L., Brokenleg, M., & Van Bockern, S. (1998). *Reclaiming Youth At Risk: Our Hope for the Future.* Bloomington, IN: National Educational Services.

APPENDICES

Appendix A

Normative Developmental Trends

Age	Cognitive Piaget	Moral Kohlberg	Psychosexual Freud	Psychosocial Erikson	Creative Lowenfeld
Infancy	Sensorimotor Birth to 2 Years		Oral Birth to 1 Year	Basic Trust vs. Mistrust Birth to 1 year Value: Hope	
Early Childhood	Pre-operational 2 to 7 Years		Anal 1 to 3 Years	Autonomy vs. Shame and Doubt 1 to 3 Years Value: Will	Scribbling Stage 2 to 4 Years
		Preconventional Stages 1. Obedience and Punishment Orientation 2. Hedonistic and Instru-mental Orientation	Phallic 3 to 6 Years	Initiative vs. Guilt 3 to 6 Years Value: Purpose	Preschematic Stage 4 to 7 Years
Childhood 7 to 11 Years	Concrete Operational	Conventional Stages 3. Good-Boy, Good-Girl Orientation 4. Authority, or Law-and-Order Orientation	Latency	Industry vs. Inferiority Values: Skill and Competence	Schematic Stage 7 to 9 Years Gang Age 9 to 12 Years
Adolescence 12 to 18 Years	Formal Operations		Genital	Identity vs. Role Confusion Value: Fidelity	Pseudo-natural-istic Stage 12 to 14 Years Adolescent Art 14 to 17 Years

Appendix B

Developmental Psychopathology: DSM-IV Classifications
Disorders Usually First Diagnosed in Infancy, Childhood, or Adolescence

Mental Retardation	Learning Disorders	Motor Skills Disorders	Communication Disorders	Pervasive Developmental Disorders
Mild Mental Retardation Moderate Mental Retardation Severe Mental Retardation Mental Retardation, Severity Unspecified	Reading Disorder Mathematics Disorder Disorder of Written Expression Learning Disorder NOS*	Developmental Coordination Disorder	Expressive Language Disorder Mixed Receptive-Expressive Language Disorder Phonological Disorder Stuttering Communication Disorder NOS*	Autistic Disorder Rett's Disorder Childhood Disintegrative Disorder Asperger's Disorder Pervasive Developmental Disorder NOS*

Attention-Deficit and Disruptive Behavior Disorders	Feeding and Eating Disorders	Tic Disorders	Elimination Disorders	Other Disorders of Infancy, Childhood, or Adolescence
Attention-Deficit/ Hyperactivity Disorder • Combined Type • Predominantly Inattentive Type • Predominantly Hyperactive-Impulsive Type Attention-Deficit/ Hyperactivity Disorder NOS* Conduct Disorder Oppositional Defiant Disorder Disruptive Behavior Disorder NOS*	Pica Rumination Disorder Feeding Disorder of Infancy or Early Childhood	Tourette's Disorder Chronic Motor or Vocal Tic Disorder Transient Tic Disorder Tic Disorder NOS*	Encopresis Enuresis	Separation Anxiety Disorder Selective Mutism Reactive Attachment Disorder of Infancy or Early Childhood Disorder of Infancy, Childhood, or Adolescence NOS*

*NOS = Not Otherwise Specified

Note. Reprinted with permission from the *Diagnostic and Statistical Manual of Mental Disorders,* Fourth Edition. Copyright 1994 by the American Psychiatric Association.

Appendix C

Psychopathology: DSM-IV Classifications

Cognitive Disorders	Substance Related Disorders	Psychotic Disorders	Mood Disorders	Anxiety Disorders	Somatoform Disorders	Factitious Disorders
Delirium Dementia Amnestic Disorders Other Cognitive Disorders	Substance Dependence Substance Abuse Substance Intoxication Substance Withdrawal	Schizophrenia Schizophreniform Disorder Schizoaffective Disorder Delusional Disorder Brief Psychotic Disorder Shared Psychotic Disorder	Depressive Disorders Bipolar Disorders	Panic Disorder Agoraphobia Specific Phobia Social Phobia Obsessive-Compulsive Disorder Posttraumatic Stress Disorder Acute Stress Disorder Generalized Anxiety Disorder	Somatization Disorder Conversion Disorder Pain Disorder Hypochondriasis Body Dysmorphic Disorder Somatoform Disorder NOS*	Factitious Disorder Factitious Disorder NOS*

Appendix C–*Continued*

Dissociative Disorders	Sexual and Gender Identity Disorders	Eating Disorders	Sleep Disorders	Impulse Control Disorders	Adjustment Disorders	Personality Disorders
Dissociative Amnesia	Sexual Dysfunction	Anorexia Nervosa	Primary Sleep Disorder	Intermittent Explosive Disorder	Adjustment Disorder	Paranoid
Dissociative Fugue	Paraphilias	Bulimia Nervosa	Sleep Disorders Related to Another Mental Disorder	Kleptomania	With Depressed Mood	Schizoid
Dissociative Identity Disorder	Gender Identity Disorders	Eating Disorder NOS*		Pyromania	With Anxiety	Schizotypal
Depersonali- zation Disorder				Pathological Gambling	With Mixed Anxiety and Depressed Mood	Antisocial
Dissociative Disorder NOS*				Trichotillo- mania	With Disturbance of Conduct	Borderline
				Impulse- Control Disorder NOS*	With Mixed Disturbance of Emotions and Conduct	Histrionic
					Unspecified	Narcissistic
						Avoidant
						Dependent
						Obsessive- Compulsive
						Personality Disorder NOS*

*NOS = Not Otherwise Specified
Note. Reprinted with permission from the *Diagnostic and Statistical Manual of Mental Disorders*, Fourth Edition. Copyright 1994 by the American Psychiatric Association.

Appendix D

Regulations of the Commissioner of Education

Pursuant to Sections 207, 3214, 4403, 4404 and 4410 of the Education Law
PART 200
Students with Disabilities
Effective January 6, 2000

200.1 Definitions.

Student with a disability means a student with a disability as defined in section 4401 (1) of Education Law, who has not attained the age of 21 prior to September 1st and who is entitled to attend public schools pursuant to section 3202 of the Education Law and who, because of mental, physical or emotional reasons, has been identified as having a disability and who requires special services and programs approved by the department. The terms used in this definition are defined as follows:

(1) *Autism* means a developmental disability significantly affecting verbal and non-verbal communication and social interaction, generally evident before age 3, that adversely affects a student's educational performance. Other characteristics often associated with autism are engagement in repetitive activities and stereotyped movements, resistance to environmental change or change in daily routines, and unusual responses to sensory experiences. The term does not apply if a student's educational performance is adversely affected primarily because the student has an emotional disturbance as defined in paragraph 4 of this subdivision. A student who manifests the characteristics of autism after age 3 could be diagnosed as having autism if the criteria in this paragraph are otherwise satisfied.

(2) *Deafness* means a hearing impairment that is so severe that the student is impaired in processing linguistic information through hearing, with or without amplification, that adversely affects a student's educational performance.

(3) *Deaf-blindness* means concomitant hearing and visual impairments, the combination of which causes such severe communication and other developmental and educational needs that they cannot be accommodated in special education programs solely for students with deafness or students with blindness.

(4) *Emotional disturbance* means a condition exhibiting one or more of the following characteristics over a long period of time and to a marked degree that adversely affects a student's educational performance:
    (i)   an inability to learn that cannot be explained by intellectual, sensory, or health factors.
    (ii) an inability to build or maintain satisfactory interpersonal relationships with peer and teachers;
    (iii) inappropriate types of behavior or feelings under normal circumstances;
    (iv) a generally pervasive mood of unhappiness or depression; or
    (v)   a tendency to develop physical symptoms or fears associated with personal or school problems.

The terms includes schizophrenia. The term does not apply to students who are socially maladjusted, unless it is determined that they have an emotional disturbance.

(5) *Hearing impairment* means an impairment in hearing, whether permanent or fluctuating, that adversely affects the child's educational performance but that is not included under the definition of *deafness* in this section.

(6) *Learning disability* means a disorder in one or more of the basic psychological processes involved in understanding or in using language, spoken or written, which manifests itself in an imperfect ability to listen, think, speak, read, write, spell, or to do mathematical calculations. The term includes such conditions as perceptual disabilities, brain injury, minimal brain dysfunction, dyslexia and developmental aphasia. The term does not include learning problems that are primarily the result of visual, hearing or motor disabilities, of mental retardation, of emotional disturbance, or of environmental, cultural or economic disadvantage. A student who exhibits a discrepancy of 50 percent or more between expected achievement and actual achievement determined on an individual basis shall be deemed to have a learning disability.

(7) *Mental retardation* means significantly subaverage general intellectual functioning, existing concurrently with deficits in adaptive behavior and manifested during the developmental period, that adversely affects a student's educational performance.

(8) *Multiple disabilities* means concomitant impairments (such as mental retardation-blindness, mental retardation-orthopedic impairment, etc.), the combination of which cause educational needs that they cannot be accommodated in a special education program solely for one of the impairments. The term does not include deaf-blindness.

(9) *Orthopedic impairment* means a severe orthopedic impairment that adversely affects a student's educational performance. The term includes impairments caused by congenital anomaly (e.g., clubfoot, absence of some member, etc.), impairments caused by disease (e.g., poliomyelitis, bone tuberculosis, etc.), and impairments from other causes (e.g., cerebral palsy, amputation, and fractures or burns which cause contractures).

(10) *Other health-impairment* means having limited strength, vitality or alertness, including a heightened alertness to environmental stimuli, that results in limited alertness with respect to the educational environment, that is due to chronic or acute health problems including but not limited to a heart condition, tuberculosis, rheumatic fever, nephritis, asthma, sickle cell anemia, hemophilia, epilepsy, lead poisoning, leukemia, diabetes, attention deficit disorder or attention deficit hyperactivity disorder or tourette syndrome, which adversely affects a student's educational performance.

(11) *Speech or language impairment* means a communication disorder, such as stuttering, impaired articulation, a language impairment or a voice impairment, that adversely affects a student's educational performance.

(12) *Traumatic brain injury* means an acquired injury to the brain caused by an external physical force or by certain medical conditions such as stroke, encephalitis, aneurysm, anoxia or brain tumors with resulting impairments that adversely affect educational performance. The term includes open or closed head injuries

or brain impairments in one or more areas, including cognition, language, memory, attention, reasoning, abstract thinking, judgement, problem solving, sensory, perceptual and motor abilities, psychosocial behavior, physical functions, information processing, and speech. The term does include injuries that are congenital or caused by birth trauma.

(13) Visual impairment including blindness means an impairment in vision that, even with correction, adversely affects a student's educational performance. The term includes both partial sight and blindness.

Note. Reprinted with permission from the Regulations of the Commissioner of Education, PART 200 – Students with Disabilities. Copyright 2000 by the State Education Department, University of the State of New York.

Appendix E

Characteristics of Successful Alternative Education Programs

School Culture	Organizational Structure	Curriculum and Instruction	System-Wide Features
Choice in Involvement: Students, teachers and staff choose to be at school; they are not placed there as a "final option." Choosing to attend the school fosters feelings of ownership and commitment to the school, facilitating a sense of community. **Focus on the Whole Student:** Alternative schools focus on personal, social, emotional, and academic development. Many programs also provide, or make available, services students may need to stay in school, such as counseling or day care. **Warm, Caring Relationships:** Warm, caring relationships with teachers are a central part of the alternative school culture. Similar relationships are also fostered in order to create a supportive peer culture. **Expanded Teacher Roles:** Teachers act not only as teachers, but also as advisors, mentors, and counselors. **Sense of Community:** Alternative programs strive to create a sense of community among teachers, staff, and students that fosters the warm, caring relationships as well as student affiliation with the school. **High Student Expectations:** Teachers have high expectations for students, but these expectations are flexible, allowing for change according to student needs.	**Small Size:** To facilitate the personal attention necessary to foster a sense of community in the alternative school, both schools and classes are small. **Relative Autonomy:** Most successful alternative education programs have some degree of freedom from standard district operating procedures. **Comprehensive Programs:** Alternative education programs include experiential learning and vocational components to link what the students learn in school with their future life and work. **Counseling:** Counseling programs are an integral part of the curriculum. They are not limited to academic issues, but help students deal with problems and events both in school and in their daily lives. **Safe Environment:** Alternative schools have a structured school environment and strict behavioral expectations that are clear to students and staff. Discipline is administered in a fair and consistent manner. **Separation from Traditional School:** Programs achieve separation either by establishing themselves in a distinct area of the traditional school or by moving to a different location entirely.	**Academic Innovation:** Programs give teachers flexibility in designing strategies and methods that will work for their students. Specific strategies include individual learning, cooperative learning, competency based learning, team teaching, peer tutoring, teaching to multiple intelligence, and an absence of tracking. Curriculum varies, ranging from programs that emphasize basic skills, to those that focus more on personal development and behavior.	**School Linked Services:** Parental involvement, community involvement, and access to basic health and social services are important features in many programs.

Note. From "Alternative Learning Environments" by Southwest Educational Development Laboratory, 1995, *INSIGHTS, No. 6.* Copyright 1995 by Southwest Educational Development Laboratory (SEDL). Reprinted with permission of Southwest Educational Development Laboratory (SEDL).

Appendix F

Sample Art Therapy Diagnostic Assessment Referral Form

Date: _____

To: _____   Title: Art Therapist

Referred By: _____   Title: _____

_____ is recommended for an Art Therapy Diagnostic

Assessment because of the following: (Please use the space below to describe any

emotional difficulties, behavior problems, or related factors that would seem

relevant.)

I feel this student may be eligible for Art Therapy because:

_____   The student often expresses him or herself through art.

_____   The student appears unable to express him or herself verbally.

_____   The student is generally withdrawn and does not appear to be a good
          candidate for verbal therapy.

_____   Art therapy adjunctive to verbal psychotherapy may be beneficial.

Appendix G

Sample Art Therapy Confidentiality Agreement

Student's Name: _____ Date:_____

I, _____ (Student), give _____

(Art Therapist), my permission to:

☐ Photograph my artwork.

☐ Duplicate my artwork.

☐ Display my artwork.

☐ Video Tape our Art Therapy session(s).

☐ Audio Tape our Art Therapy session(s).

☐ Use my artwork in research, teaching, writing, and public presentations.

☐ Use our session dialogue in research, teaching, writing, and public presentations.

I understand that in all cases, _____ (Art Therapist) will take

appropriate steps to protect my identity. If at any time I choose to withdraw my

permission, I will contact this Art Therapist and my request will be honored imme-

diately. I understand that for research and/or writing purposes my withdrawal of

permission cannot be grandfathered.

Signed: _____(Student)

Signed: _____(Parent/Guardian)

Signed: _____(Art Therapist)

Note. Revised with permission from Jill Penaloza.

INDEX